Dear Body

ALSO BY BRITTANY WILLIAMS

Instant Loss Cookbook
Instant Loss: Eat Real, Lose Weight
Instant Loss on a Budget

Dear Body

WHAT I LOST,
WHAT I GAINED,
and WHAT I LEARNED
ALONG THE WAY

BRITTANY WILLIAMS

Creator of **Instant Loss**

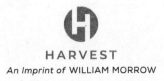

HARVEST
An Imprint of WILLIAM MORROW

Some names and identifying details have been changed.

HarperCollins books may be purchased for educational, business, or sales promotional use. For information, please email the Special Markets Department at SPsales@harpercollins.com.

FIRST EDITION

Designed by Renata DiBiase

Library of Congress Cataloging-in-Publication Data has been applied for.

ISBN 978-0-358-53991-9

22 23 24 25 26 LBC 5 4 3 2 1

Dear Body,

Life has often felt full of conflict. I've felt dissonance in body, being, and self. There has been grief, shame, and affliction but also deep love, immense joy, and persistent hope, always hope. It seeps through every crack and crevice, bubbling up, spilling out into even the darkest of moments, undeniable.

Living in this body is both a sacred and complicated experience. I promise to stay open, willing, and present as we continue to make our way through the world together.

Our relationship is complex and ever changing: That's what makes it beautiful.

Contents

Contents

A Story

Dear Body,
    Today I promise to honor you with intention.

Ring.

My foot jittered involuntarily, my neon-orange toenails tracing an invisible line on the floor as I cradled my cell phone on my shoulder, listening to it ring on the other end. I'd had restless legs syndrome since I was a preteen; today it felt less like a nuisance and more like anticipation.

My hands were occupied, holding my nine-month-old as he nursed distractedly, latching, then pulling off to laugh at his siblings. The older kids were playing on the floor with an array of wooden cooking spoons, pots, and old containers. They preferred to play with the items we used every day rather than the buckets of toys that littered their rooms. Go figure.

Ring.

I sighed and shifted my position on our old leather hand-me-down couch. I caught a whiff of the cinnamon streusel banana bread baking in the oven. It smelled like autumn, although it was March, and I made a mental note to check it after my phone call. Was it so irrational to want my mom to answer my calls on the first ring?

Life had been full lately and I had a feeling that this fullness was about to expand. My excitement always began to build in the springtime and blossomed fully in the summer when the weather got hot and the sun shone brightest. But this was different. This was a new kind of energy. My spirit was nearly shouting that I was on the precipice of something. My gut was telling me to go, build, make—but my brain was quick to remind me that I had three children under five and that all of my attention should be focused on them.

Ring.

But I couldn't shake this feeling that I should be doing something more. I thought of my aunt Kim, who always said that your identity should never be so wrapped up in your children that you didn't know who you were anymore when they left. *You're not raising children,* I could practically hear her voice in my mind, *you're raising adults.* I knew that it was just as important for me to invest in and take care of myself as it was for me to care for them. Maybe even a little more important. As the saying goes, you can't pour from an empty cup.

Just a few months earlier—January 4, 2017, to be exact—I had decided to practice intentionality when it came to filling that cup. And it was Aunt Kim's words that assuaged my societally conditioned mom guilt when I began to take moments for myself. For the first time in my life, I realized it was necessary to cultivate a lifestyle that encouraged my long-term health and wellness. There was a meme that had been floating around the internet that said *We would all die for our children, but are we willing to live for them?* I wanted to live for my children, but I was discovering how important it was to live for myself.

Ring.

Actually live. Make positive choices that supported longevity and sanctity of mind, body, and spirit. This was something big for me. Soul-rattling, person-changing. A revelation that practicing self-love with nothing but a massage, pedicure, or bubble bath wasn't the type of care that my mind, body, and spirit truly needed. What I really needed was the courage to dig deep below the surface and uncover the roots of the illness that had kept me from reaching my full potential, that I had so carefully buried over the years because facing it was too much to bear.

But I was twenty-seven now and responsible for mothering these three beautiful little beings, and I knew that unhealed trauma, no matter how deeply buried, always rises to the surface, begging to be dealt with. So I greeted 2017 with a goal to heal, and as I became diligent about taking time for my own health and wellness, I began to feel like it all might be for some greater, grander, more extraordinary purpose than I had ever imagined.

Ring—

"Hellooo." My mom's musical voice practically sang through the other end.

"Well, hello to you!" I responded with a smile. We worked through our usual niceties— "What have you been up to?" "How's Dad?" "How are the kids?"—before she cut to the chase.

"What's up?"

"Have you ever felt like something's coming? Something big and inexplicably life-changing, but you can't figure out what it is and why you feel that way and you don't know if it's really a premonition or just last night's lasagna?" I asked all in one breath. My mom chuckled softly as I sat the baby on the floor with his siblings.

"Hmm," she murmured. "Off the top of my head, I can't say that I have. Is there something you want to be doing?" I heard her fiddling in the background and guessed she probably had me on speakerphone as she worked through one of her paint-by-numbers on her favorite iPhone app.

I went to go check on my banana bread. "I feel like I'm supposed to be doing something more."

She hmmed again and asked me how my challenge was going. She knew that my New Year's resolution was to invest more time into cooking. Starting in January, I had challenged myself to cook dinner at home every night with real, minimally processed or unprocessed foods. If there was a party or function we had to attend, we could eat out, as long as I stuck to real food. In other words, I'd eat stuff that came from the earth, not a laboratory. I'd spent the past six years researching ingredients and educating myself about the importance of what goes into the body—and on it. By making small changes over time, I'd been able to see the benefits that came from being mindful about these things.

But what I really wanted to focus on was managing my time better so we could eat this way every day, not just some days. As a stay-at-home mom, I knew I could find the time to make meals if I reorganized my life a little. Up until that point, I'd fallen stomach-first into having the hubs pick up dinner several nights a week on his way home—pizza, Taco Bell, and the occasional Wendy's drive-through had turned into our normal routine instead of something we resorted to in a pinch. I knew that the food choices we were making didn't support a healthy lifestyle, and I was on a mission to change that.

I opened the oven and stuck a toothpick in the loaf of banana bread; it was perfect. I pulled it out and set it on a wire rack to cool. "It's going really well. I've lost forty-six pounds in three months. My doctor told me to stop taking my Synthroid because, for the first time in ten years, my thyroid was *over*medicated. She thinks that I may have reversed my thyroid disease."

"That's fantastic!" she said.

"I know. I think about all of those people out there in the world who have accepted sickness as their baseline. I didn't even realize how sick I was until I felt better. I find myself saying constantly, 'I can't believe how good I feel.' Because the truth is, I was sick, but I lived with it for so long, I forgot how it felt not to be sick. And now that I'm healing and recognizing how important ingredients are, I want to shout it from the rooftops!" I punctuated that statement with a bang of my spatula as I tidied up the counter from my baking.

"You might be onto something," my mom said. "You should pray about it."

"I've been hearing that a lot lately." And I had. Every time I discussed this feeling with my husband, he was adamant that prayer was the answer. I was reminded of one of my kids' favorite movies, *Frozen,* and I felt like Elsa, full of excitement and trepidation, on the precipice of launching herself into the unknown.

That afternoon I prayed about the nagging mystical stirrings, and I kept praying about them anytime they surfaced. And then, two weeks later, on a regular Tuesday afternoon while my husband was away on a five-day work trip, and I was solo-mom-ing, it hit me smack in the face. At the time, I didn't realize exactly what that "it" meant, but at that moment, I knew I'd launched myself off the precipice and into the uncharted territory of the beyond. Beyond myself. Beyond my doing. Beyond the limitations of my imagination.

I wrote a random post in a Facebook group about eating healthy while breastfeeding, and it went viral. Before I knew it, I had a group of people who wanted to know how I'd lost so much weight in such a short time. My rapid weight loss hooked them and made my story "newsworthy" and appealing. But it was never about the weight loss for me; that was just what got my foot in the door and allowed me to tell the story I really wanted to tell. The one about how I felt condemned to live a life within a body that felt like a prison cell instead of a reflection of who I truly was. A story about how making small but calculated choices—on everything from what I ate to how I approached my relationships—coalesced into true transformation. A story about how I once was sick but now am healed.

1

Becoming

Dear Body,
   Thank you for being the vessel that carries all
of my thoughts, dreams, and hopes for the future.
Thank you for supporting me in my adventures then,
now, and always.

When I was really young, my parents bought me a little tape player/recorder. It was white with a handle, two big black eyes, and a big red smile where you inserted the tape, and a bright yellow spiral cord that ended in a microphone. I ruled the world with that microphone, let me tell you. I was a force to be reckoned with, bossing around my little brothers and sister at only six years old while singing about ladybugs, the sky, and fantastical imaginary things.

   Weekends were spent on a makeshift stage in our front yard. Built out of discarded cardboard boxes, sheets, and blankets, with flashlights for spotlights, it was the perfect place to put on dramatic performances for the neighborhood kids. Fearless, I sang and danced my way across the cardboard-covered grass. Microphone in one hand and baton in the other, I was blissfully oblivious to anyone else's opinions as I sashayed and improvised words to music that only I could hear. I would tumble, twirl, and sing—and, thankfully, the other kids would clap and cheer. Like Tinker Bell, I needed applause to live.

When no one could come out to play—which meant I had no audience—I would perform for the big sweet gum tree in our front yard or I'd watch my reflection in our living-room window. Sometimes, if I squeezed my eyes closed tightly and opened them real quick, I'd be transported from our Southern California cul-de-sac to a stage in a palace full of royals or to the deck of a fancy cruise ship or to the lights of Broadway. There were no limits to where I could go or what I could do.

When I was in first grade, my mom signed me up for the school talent show. She sat with me in her bathroom the night before and carefully sectioned my long brown hair, then rolled it up in light pink sponge curlers. The day of the show she did my makeup; it was the first time I'd ever worn any, and it made me feel so grown up. She bought me a special outfit for the occasion, a blue denim dress with a black cowboy hat.

Backstage in the auditorium, I remember experiencing an unnerving feeling. My stomach was all balled up and heavy, and my face felt both hot and cold at the same time. "I don't feel so good, Mom," I told her.

"You're probably just a little nervous. You'll do great!" She kissed me on the forehead and left to find her seat.

Nervous. I'd never been nervous before, but thinking about all of those real live people with all of their real live eyes on me was making my heart speed up. What if I forgot the words? What if I messed up? For the first time, I began to doubt myself. I looked around the room at all the other performers. Our school ran from elementary to high school, so most of them were much older than I was. A high-school boy caught my eye; I'm sure he recognized the deer-in-the-headlights look on my face. "Hey, I heard you at practice the other day," he said, approaching me and bending down to my eye level. "Everyone is going to be amazed that someone so little has such a big voice."

I barely had time to say "Thank you" before one of the teachers called my name and said I was up next. My palms were sweating around the microphone, and I began to feel like I really shouldn't be doing this—that maybe I was too young, too little. But the second I stepped onto that stage, every nerve I had melted away into supernatural calmness. The bright lights of the auditorium blinded my eyes, and I was transported back to that piece of cardboard in my front yard as I took a deep breath, smiled brightly, and began to sing.

"'Phone rings, baby cries, TV diet guru lies.'" "XXX's and OOO's" by Trisha Yearwood was my favorite song and I felt like a star as I belted out the lyrics with confidence. Everything felt heightened. More intense. More real. More right. It was before I was able to name that feeling, but my gut recognized it right away: it was euphoria. And every show, every performance I did—even ones where I wasn't on a stage in front of hundreds or, sometimes, thousands of people—was my attempt at prolonging it, bottling it up so I'd never have to go without it. When I was performing, it was like I was doing exactly what I was made to do, living inside a perfect moment, a feeling that comes only when you are doing what you know you were created for.

My parents always supported my desire to be on the stage. My mom signed me up for dance classes, and I even got to walk in a fashion show arranged by her work. She never missed a performance or an opportunity to tell me how proud she was. "You're very special and very talented," she would say. "I don't know any other little girls who can do all of the things that you can do." And I believed her. I *believed* that I was special.

As I grew up and matured, performing began to take a back seat to all the responsibilities that tend to take precedence over dreams. One of the hardest things about life is that everything changes. Ironically, it's also one of the most beautiful things about it. We'll reinvent ourselves a hundred times, chasing euphoria because we know it exists and trying to reconcile who we were with who we are becoming.

2

Innocence

Dear Body,
   Here's what I have learned over time: Other
people's ideas and opinions about you belong to
them. I didn't always know this, but I promise to
shield you from negativity by affirming you with
truth from now on.

I remember a time when all I felt was promise, and everything came easily. I fit in at school, got along with others,
was viewed as someone exceptional and uncommon. People
seemed drawn to me—teachers responded to me, adults encouraged me, and I felt from the beginning like I was going to
do big things and have a big impact on the world.

   I didn't think much about my body back then. My time
was better spent performing concerts in our empty cul-de-sac,
dreaming about singing, dancing, and inhabiting castles in
kingdoms. Staying out until the streetlights came on, sending
my siblings and me home. I believed that I could achieve or

receive anything life had to offer. I was young, innocent, and completely unspoiled by the potential heartache the world could bring. That naïveté was beautiful.

Food fueled my body for the activities that filled my day. It allowed me to perform and play and keep up with the very busy life I was leading. We were one, my body and I, completely in sync, and I had much greater things to think and dream about.

And then things changed. I remember the first time I thought about my body as something separate, something negative.

It was my younger brother Connor's eighth birthday. We had a swim party for him in August. I was only fourteen. It was chaos—kids running around, food on every surface, our big extended family squeezing into a little house, filling every nook and cranny. I remember walking into the house, still dripping from the pool, a bright orange towel around my shoulders that matched the dark orange flowers of my bathing suit.

As I headed to the counter, I inhaled the delicious smell of barbecue and tried not to let my wet feet slip on the kitchen tile. We had already eaten lunch, but I wanted a handful or two of Cheetos, my favorite snack, and maybe a cup of root beer or Mountain Dew. I started to fill a plate with snacks when the towel around me fell to the ground, and family members squeezed by me in the kitchen.

My stepgrandma knelt down to pick up my towel. As she handed it to me, she said in her thick Mexican accent, "You need to learn how to hold in your tummy."

"Huh?" I asked, sure I hadn't heard her right.

"My mother taught me, and someone needs to teach you. You need to squeeze your tummy and hold it in." She looked down at my plate. "You also shouldn't eat those things anymore. You are becoming a woman now, and no man will want you with a pudgy figure like that."

"Okay," I muttered. My demeanor changed instantly. I wrapped my towel around my body self-consciously, abandoned my Cheetos on the counter, lowered my head, and retreated to my bedroom. For the next several minutes, I stood in front of my full-length mirror, Gwen Stefani staring at me from the poster above my bed. First, I practiced sucking in my stomach. Then I poked at it, wondering why I had never realized how soft and squishy it was. It had ripples and dimples; those weren't supposed to be there? I knew I'd recently developed stretch marks on my sides, but my mom had those too. Weren't they just beauty marks that showed I was developing into a woman?

I continued to study myself. I wasn't preening or admiring; I was evaluating, judging my body for the first time based on someone else's standard. It was like a veil had been lifted from my eyes and the truth was suddenly coming to light. My consciousness floated above my head, looking down on my body: thighs too big, tummy too soft, bottom too round.

Now it was like the floodgates had opened and comments that had once fallen on deaf, uncaring ears were ringing loudly, like the sounding of a gong.

"Certainly not the body of a dancer," I'd heard someone whisper before.

"You have such a pretty face," I could hear one of my aunts say. Now that I thought about it, it seemed that many people had made a point of admiring just my face instead of simply stating, "I think you're pretty."

I remembered one of the theater moms making a big deal about how I couldn't wear the same costume as my counterpart in the performance because I was a size bigger, and they'd have to buy another. And many boys at school had commented on how big my butt was. I'd laughed, thinking it was a joke, but now I realized it wasn't a joke at all.

I couldn't share clothes with my friends or my sister. One of my aunts had told me that I was good enough to win *American Idol* . . . if I lost twenty-five pounds.

I stared harder in the mirror and squeezed my tummy between my fingers. I pulled on it, remembering a girl at school telling me that if I could pinch more than an inch, it meant that I was fat. What did it mean if I was able to grab a handful?

It was true, then.

I was fat.

When had that even happened?

As I stared, I remembered that Mom and Dad had just started that new SlimFast diet. Maybe I could eat a bar or drink a shake or two? I was sure just a small change would do the trick. I knew Mom still had some Metabolife pills, and Dad was taking an appetite suppressant—if SlimFast didn't work, maybe I could sneak some of those too.

I'd seen my parents try diet after diet in an attempt to lose weight, everything from doctor-prescribed pills to the Hollywood juice diet. And though nothing ever really seemed to work for them, I thought that maybe it would work for me. In an instant, my body-neutral stance shifted into an all-out war.

Lose twenty-five pounds, my inner voice whispered. *You can pinch more than an inch.* My inner voice began to sound suspiciously like my stepgrandma's. *No one will want you with a pudgy figure like that.* Pandora's box had been opened, and there was no going back. I wasn't upset; I wondered why I'd never listened to those voices before. Why hadn't I taken action before it got so out of hand? And now, even though I hadn't realized it was happening, it was clear that it was my fault and my obligation to do something about it.

I knew my stepgrandma hadn't meant to hurt my feelings or cause me to doubt myself—she thought she was doing me a favor, passing down valuable information, woman to woman. But my life up until that point had been focused only on expanding, growing, unlocking all the world had to offer. As I stood sideways, sucking my tummy in as far as it would go, I began to think about shrinking, diminishing, lessening.

I don't believe that we are born doubting ourselves, our bodies, or our worth. I believe we are born the headliners, the stars of our own shows. But there are little, seemingly innocuous things that happen throughout our lives that begin to change us. Sometimes we unintentionally invite this into our lives or permit it because of the people we let get in our heads. People who use their words to discourage or bring us down instead of to empower and uplift. Unfortunately, their words add up; they become thoughts we attribute to our own shortcomings. Today I know my stepgrandma was speaking from a place of her own pain—her mother had told her to make herself smaller, and she passed that message on to me. I internalized her message. I let her words take hold, dim my spotlight, eat away at my confidence, and distort my self-image.

Innocence lost.

The good news is that our innocence, our self-love, isn't gone for good; it just needs to be found again. Our bodies are the one thing that will always be with us, from the time we're born to the time we leave this earth. I was proud of my body, and then I wasn't, and it's taken me a really long time to be proud of it once again. But what matters is that I got there. And if I got there, you can too.

3

Cure-All

Dear Body,

It's hard when the people who are supposed to protect you are the ones you need protection from. It's confusing to experience such harshness and such great love all at once. When food is used to buy silence, soothe wounds, and bring comfort in addition to celebrate, bond, and nourish, it can create unhealthy behaviors or coping mechanisms. Emotional eating was something we discovered when we were young. Food was used for convenience, happiness, apologies, and it became my favorite form of avoidance.

Human emotion is incredibly complex. We are multidimensional beings, capable of feeling a plethora of emotions all at once, even ones that are difficult to reconcile with one another.

On the one hand, I had the best childhood I could imagine; on the other, it was a complicated quagmire of conflicting events and reactions. The kindest things my parents ever said to me are tempered by my memories of the worst. We talked about everything except for the topics we weren't allowed to talk about: the fighting, the physical abuse, the verbal assaults.

My parents were very young when they got married; my mom is just barely eighteen years my senior. My six siblings followed me in quick succession. Practically overnight, my parents went from two kids in puppy love to full-blown adults with an overwhelming amount of responsibility. Being so close in age to my parents, I felt like they were my best friends; they always supported everything I did, and I could talk to them about almost anything, from performance critiques to boy troubles. We rode roller coasters together, went on Slurpee dates, and they drove me to every voice, dance, gymnastics, cheer, and piano lesson without complaint.

But there was a lot of emotional immaturity in their relationship with each other and with their kids. There were shouting matches, slamming doors; there was name-calling and vindictive behavior. Anything—and especially those things that were important to someone—could be weaponized; they fought dirty, both verbally and physically. There was fierce fighting, but there was also fierce love. And the contrast was confusing.

I assumed this was the way all families functioned behind closed doors.

Sprawled out on a towel in my backyard with my friend Amanda, I decided to ask her the question that was frequently at the forefront of my mind. "Do your parents ever fight?"

She had been taking a swig of her diet cola and spluttered a bit. "Do my parents fight?" she asked sarcastically. "That's like asking if the sky is blue—of course they do."

I chuckled a little and rolled onto my tummy. "Yeah, everyone fights, right? But I mean like screaming, cussing, throwing things, Mom-leaving-and-saying-she's-never-going-to-come-back kind of fights. Like: Steer clear, everybody, or you're liable to be collateral damage. Fight-fights."

Amanda sighed and set her soda down on the grass. She tucked her legs underneath her before saying in a hushed voice, "My parents are crazy, so I'm probably not the one to ask if you want the gauge for 'normal'"—she air-quoted the word. "But yeah, things get nasty. My dad pushed me down the stairs because he didn't like the shorts I was going to wear to school." She extended her leg and pointed to a yellowing bruise.

I parted my hair to uncover a scabbed cut on my head. "Laptop computer."

She nodded. "I'm not saying it's right, but I love them and they love me, and it's better than being in foster care until I'm eighteen."

I nodded too, remembering the morning after the laptop altercation.

I'd come out of my bedroom to find Mom dancing in front of the stove and making stacks of pancakes. "Morning, Brit!" she'd said. "I hope you slept well! Today is gonna be so much fun!"

I slid into a chair at the table and stared at her. I knew my family well enough to realize the intense drama from the night before would be swept under the rug. My dad walked into the room and nodded at me. "Morning, Spit! Let's skip school today. We'll all hang out here—order some pizza, grab some snacks from Walmart, root-beer-float it up, and watch movies! We'll start the weekend early!"

I smiled as my siblings exclaimed, "That sounds awesome!"

My dad served himself as I sliced into the pancakes and slid the sweet, buttery bite into my mouth. The deep, salty butter, the fluff of the pancake, the stinging sweetness of the syrup—to me, they all translated to love. And a veg-out day, as our family called it, was an entire day full of delicious, comforting, heartwarming love that often followed a hard day, a tumultuous night, or a fight that didn't end well. My parents would pile us into the van, and we'd go to every fast-food restaurant in town, ordering absolutely anything we wanted. Then we'd come home, draw the curtains, and watch silly movies and funny TV shows all day long. If we had school, we'd skip it. If they had work, they'd call in sick. This was how we healed. Not with reassuring, apologetic words but with food and entertainment.

Hours later, I sat in the middle of a king-size blanket on the floor of the family room, the light from the TV forming a soft aura around the nine of us. I bit into a greasy cheeseburger, chased it with warm, salty fries, then washed everything down with a frigid chocolate milkshake so thick, it almost wouldn't travel up the straw. As the actor on-screen delivered a famous punch line, the room erupted in laughter. I leaned forward, trying not to spit my milkshake across the room. My sister nudged my leg and we exchanged smiles. In that moment, my sadness deeply buried beneath a layer of delicious food, the pain from the day before vanished, and all was right again with the world.

Parents never start out with the intent to harm their children. Now that I'm a mother, I can understand how tough my parents had it. Kids aren't born with a guidebook or owner's manual showing you how to parent. My parents are human—sometimes they made poor choices, sometimes they made *wrong* choices, but my God, how they *tried*.

Trauma and abuse were part of my childhood, but they weren't the only part. All told, the good memories far outweigh the bad ones, but the bad ones are still there. Just like good memories, they have shaped the person I'm becoming.

When I look back on my childhood, I see several lessons I learned that I carried with me into adulthood. First: Complex emotions should be avoided, buried, and not discussed. Second: Admitting personal wrongdoing is damaging, and when you're wrong, it's better to cling to justifications than to admit you've made a mistake. Third: Apologizing for your poor behavior is humiliating; you can expect that from others, but apologies evoke too many feelings of vulnerability, inadequacy, and incompetence to ever utter yourself.

And, finally: Food is the ultimate cure-all.

4

Food and Fantasy

Dear Body,
   For years, I struggled to learn how to cope with
my feelings and emotions in positive, healthy ways.
Growing up, I found comfort in food and dealt with
tough feelings by avoiding them instead of facing
them. In this way, I unintentionally abused you. I still
haven't healed those parts of me entirely yet, but I'm
working on it.

I shuffled upstairs to my bedroom, tossed my purse onto a
chair, made my way around the scattered piles of clothes,
shoes, and books on the floor, and launched myself onto the
bed. Aside from the glowing lamp on my bedside table,
the only light in the room came from my computer screen—
the brightness fading each time my *Buffy the Vampire Slayer*
screen saver flipped to a new image. I was barely sixteen and
had just scored my first job as a hostess at Mimi's Café. Things
were going well so far; I was meeting new people, making new

friends. Work seemed less like work and more like an escape into the adult world I wanted to live in so badly but wasn't quite ready for yet.

Buffy gazed out from the screen, her stance wide; she was gripping a stake, claiming her space, radiating confidence. My mind wandered as I laid back, hair spilling across my pillow, and imagined a fairy-tale scenario. I closed my eyes and made believe that I was at the Bronze in Sunnydale with friends, my secret identity as a superhero vampire slayer hidden beneath my hot pink tube top and black leather miniskirt. I could dance and slay demons equally well, a beguiling and dangerous combination . . .

I flipped over onto my stomach, and my black Dickies work pants pinched my tummy.

"Ugh." I sighed as I popped the button and let the zipper down a little bit. I noticed the indentations my pants had left on my stomach over the course of the workday. *The pants must have shrunk in the wash,* I thought; I had bought them a couple of weeks ago when I started working at Mimi's. Surely I couldn't have gone up a size already. I had been taking advantage of the free-for-employees soup, salad, and bread perk, but I hadn't been eating *that* much, had I? Uncomfortable and frustrated that a trip to the store to buy another thirty-dollar pair of pants was in my future, I shimmied out of them and kicked them off, giving them a good hard glare in the process. I was certainly no demon huntress or mysterious dance-floor beauty.

There was no way I could ever rock outfits like the girls on TV; miniskirts and halter tops were not part of my wardrobe. Although that wasn't just because I didn't think they would flatter my figure. My parents had pretty strict rules about what I was and was not allowed to wear, rules that I understood and respected but sometimes resented. I wanted to be beautiful and coveted, like the heroines on TV, the pop stars in magazines, and the models in the *Sports Illustrated* Swimsuit Issue that my dad confiscated from my brother but let me have since I liked to look at the pretty suits. But I didn't really fit that mold. My sister did; my friends did. I couldn't even get my size 15 Dickies to cooperate.

I remembered a conversation I'd had with my aunt Kim a few days earlier. Married to my mom's younger brother, she'd been in my life since I was two and was my go-to person for advice. Like a cool older sister, she was always there to listen and direct me through the storms of life. I often had a difficult time deciphering my feelings. I grew up in an era where phrases like *tough love, suck it up,* and *get over it* were staples for parenting, and that didn't exactly foster healthy coping mechanisms. Instead of feeling my feelings, I was encouraged to push them away, and I learned how to bury them in food, friends, escapism—like reading lots of fiction and watching reruns of Sarah Michelle Gellar verbally and physically sparring with monsters and villains—even songwriting. Aunt Kim helped ground me and she talked me through the ever-present conflict within myself: to feel or not to feel. There was no one I admired or looked up to more.

During this particular conversation, we were chatting about the family fun we'd had over the holidays. "I feel like if I ate one more piece of pumpkin pie, I might burst!" I exclaimed.

She chuckled softly and commiserated. "Girlfriend, I tried on my cute-butt jeans the other night, and I couldn't even get them to button."

"Cute-butt jeans?" I asked.

"You know! The ones you said make me look like I'm a cool mom because of the holes in the knees?" I did remember; I envied those jeans. I wasn't allowed to buy jeans with holes in them—my parents thought they were a waste—but man, oh, man, did Aunt Kim look awesome in them.

"You call them cute-butt jeans?" I laughed. "I love that!"

"Every girl has got to have at least one pair of cute-butt jeans—it's the rules. It just sucks when the pie catches up with you and they don't look so cute anymore," she said wistfully.

Thinking about this, after having just flung my far-from-cute too-tight work pants on the floor, I felt a little jolt of inspiration. I began to hum a melody as I reached over and grabbed a pen off my nightstand and a stray envelope that had once held a paycheck. I flipped it over and started to scribble: *When your cute-butt jeans are a little too tight, honey, that's life—*

Songwriting was a safe place for me to process emotions and let my imagination run wild. I'd spend hours locked up in my room in front of my electronic keyboard with a composition notebook, the windows open wide as I penned lyrics about love, longing, heartbreak, and life. Most were subjects I'd never experienced but desperately wanted to.

I cast a dark look at those binding, pinching, dumb black pants bunched up on the floor and my hand started to fly—

Cute-Butt Jeans

Woke up today, half past ten
The alarm clock is broken again
And I'm wondering if my car's gonna start today

Have to work on Saturday
A stack of bills I forgot to pay
And I'm fishing change out of the cushions of my seat

Life has got to get better
There has to be more than this
Getting by but I won't lie, it's harder than I
*   anticipated*

Don't you hate it when your hair looks cute and it
starts to rain?
Don't you hate it when your nails feel dry and
*   smudge anyway?*
Don't you hate it when your cute-butt jeans are a
*   little too tight?*

Honey, that's life.

Don't you hate it when you gain ten pounds' worth
of holiday?
Don't you hate it when you get a late fee 'cause
*   you're one day late?*
Don't you hate it when your cute-butt jeans are a
*   little too tight?*

Honey, that's life!

I punctuated my new little ditty with an exclamation point and grabbed the phone to call Aunt Kim and share my new song. Who needed miniskirts anyway?

If I was honest with myself, I knew it wasn't just the bottomless bread bowls at Mimi's that were to blame. When I wasn't writing songs to process my emotions, I turned to food. And, unfortunately, that food left *a lot* to be desired.

When I was growing up, the USDA food pyramid was the

gold standard, the eating guide they taught us in school. The bottom and widest part of the pyramid featured carbohydrates, like bread and potatoes; above that were fruits and veggies; above that, sharing a level, was dairy—like milk and cheese—and meat; and finally, at the very top, fats, like butter and oil. The idea was that your daily food intake should mimic the pattern outlined by the pyramid: Eat more carbohydrates, plenty of fruits and veggies, moderate amounts of dairy and meat, and minimal fats.

Today, healthy-eating experts advise you to shop the outside aisles of the grocery store, to focus on greens, fruits, and weird-sounding things, like good bacteria, and to minimize processed foods. But in the 1990s, we hadn't figured any of that out yet, and most families gravitated toward food that was convenient: pizza rolls, Chef Boyardee, Top Ramen, and Kool-Aid. Women on diets ate frozen, processed lean meals and one-hundred-calorie ultra-processed snacks; they focused on Weight Watchers points. Liquid diets made it possible to drink chocolate shakes for every meal and still get skinny. We didn't think it was weird at the time, but let's face it: If something sounds too good to be true, it probably is.

My family was no different. Like many, we were oblivious to the importance of healthy food. I don't think we could have told you what healthy was. My parents were crash-dieters who tried any diet that was trendy at the time. The kids cobbled together meals that could be made quickly—usually cupboard snacks, cereal, hot dogs, frozen burritos, or bags of frozen French fries warmed up by yours truly. As the oldest of seven, I was responsible for many things most other children were not: changing diapers, making meals for my siblings, even warming breast milk to bottle-feed the baby in the middle of the night when my mom worked the night shift.

I took on that responsibility early and with pride. Though it wasn't long before I was confronted with the truth that this wasn't necessarily the way most families functioned, it was how we operated. For better or worse.

My dad was on medical disability, and my mom was a nurse who worked the graveyard shift. This often left the oldest kids responsible for the youngest. I've always said that I've been a mom my whole life. I had to grow up quickly because those around me needed me to be more than a big sister when my mom wasn't there.

I didn't realize until I became an adult that it was during these years that I began to use food to soothe and comfort myself. It was a response born out of watching my parents try to heal their trauma and discomfort with food and avoidance—something that became as natural to me as breathing. I'd spend hours tucked away in my room writing about fictional characters who were living idealized lives; I corrected situations in fantasy that I couldn't fix in reality.

It would take years for me to realize that escaping into fiction and food, once a survival mechanism, became an unhealthy stranglehold. I'd lose days shut up in my room reading and writing when I was supposed to be doing other things. This coping device began to affect my grades, my work schedule, and my social life. Reading and writing aren't inherently negative, but I allowed them to consume my every waking moment. There were long periods when I didn't want to exist within the real world because the fantasy was so much better.

Turning to food for comfort is incredibly common; it's probably one of the earliest coping mechanisms people develop. Most of us can trace it back to our mothers and breastfeeding. Comforting yourself with food is not always harmful—there's something to be said for the warm feeling you get when you gather with family and friends and eat traditional foods during holidays—but it's a problem when it's your only way of handling your feelings, and it grew out of control in my life. I went from using food for solace to using it when I felt bored, excited, sad—any emotion was an excuse to eat. This became my vice, food my drug of choice—and it was a socially acceptable one.

The real problem wasn't that I was addicted to food; it was that I had never learned how to emote in positive ways and that I felt helpless to adapt to change. I was overwhelmed, depressed, and dissatisfied, but it was easier to just say, "I'm hungry," than to deal with all of that. This had a sweeping and debilitating effect on my life in the years to come in ways I could never have imagined.

5

Immodest

Dear Body,

There was a time when it cut deeply when people criticized us for what we wore or how we looked in an attempt to get us to fall in line and conform to a certain standard. People can be unrelenting in their judgment, and some take pleasure in throwing rocks at things that shine. But now I know that dressing the way I want to is not a trespass against God. In fact, it's a trespass against ourselves if we don't explore our creative freedom.

What I wore was often a bone of contention in my family, largely because of my shape; I have always been a curvy girl. I was a little bit of a fashionista—I liked to wear the latest trends, and I looked up to style icons like Gwen Stefani, Cher from *Clueless,* and Britney Spears. But growing up in a conservative family, I was not allowed to wear crop tops, spaghetti straps, short skirts, or low-cut jeans. While I understood that my parents had my best interests in mind, I couldn't help but wonder what the harm was in wearing a crop top every once in a while. After all, boys could wear pretty much whatever they wanted.

It seemed that adults and authorities everywhere had one set of rules for boys and one for girls. The dress code for girls filled an entire page in the school handbook; the boys' dress code was only a paragraph long. The school dictated how long girls' shorts, skirts, and dresses needed to be and even how we wore our hair. Bleached hair was okay but you couldn't have any unnatural colors. Hairstyles had to be traditional—no mohawks or dreadlocks—and you couldn't wear hats or bandannas.

In the 1990s, it was super-trendy for boys to spike their hair and bleach the tips blond; popular boy bands sported the look. My brothers rocked this style. It was popular for girls to bleach the ends of their hair and dye about two inches of the bottom in fun colors. The summer before I started seventh grade, after months of pleading, my mom took me to the salon so I could get my hair styled this way. I had them dye the tips red, and I was thrilled beyond belief. She reminded me that she would have to cut the ends off at the end of the summer. When it came time for school to start again, I begged my mom not to cut it. She warned me that I would probably get sent home, but she let me go to school that way.

I made it to third period before I was sent to the assistant principal's office. He informed me that if I wanted to continue coming to school, I had to cut off the ends of my hair, because hair dyeing was against the girls' dress code. When I asked why the boys were allowed to color their hair but the girls were not, the assistant principal said that if girls colored their hair, it could distract other children from learning. I told him that I felt the rules were infringing on my right to freedom of expression. (I was a feisty little thing.) I went on to explain that my hair was less of a hindrance to learning than keeping me from class was.

He smiled a little, amused, as I spoke. Then he informed me that by attending public school, I had relinquished my rights of freedom of expression and freedom of speech, and he gave me two days of lunchtime detention for breaking the dress code. As I was leaving, he told me candidly and "off the record" that he thought the rule was stupid too, and he liked my moxie.

I am not proposing we abolish all dress codes; I understand that there are times and places that call for a certain standard of dress, and because women have so many more options, there will inherently be more regulation. But as a young woman, I found it incredibly frustrating to continuously come up against different codes of dress and conduct—at home, at church, and at school—just because I was a girl. It didn't help that my younger sister didn't seem to face the same restrictions in her smaller, less curvy body. Thinner girls often face less scrutiny than girls who are more curvaceous when it comes to dress, even in something as simple as a baby-doll T-shirt and shorts. There is a certain adultification that comes with being plus-size or more filled out—having bigger breasts, a curvier waist, a rounder bottom; it garners more attention, regardless of what one wears. My sister could wear shorts and a tank top and look entirely wholesome, but I'd wear the same outfit and judgmental eyes would find me. Like I was purposefully trying to evoke an illicit response. While I dreamed of rebelling against the rules, I largely abided by them; it was the easiest course of action, and I didn't want to have a daily battle over how I looked or what I wore.

Looking back on it now, I realize I gave up fighting the rules only to turn against my body; the only fight I faced was one within myself. If only my body were less curvaceous. If only I had smaller boobs, took up less space, could fit into a size small. If only I could conform to the model of a girl that the schools, churches, and authority figures were trying to create, I wouldn't have this inner battle raging over what was allowed and what I felt was right.

As I got older, I recognized that a lot of this body- and style-policing stemmed from a place of fear—fear that girls who wore certain clothes, dressed a certain way, or even colored their hair would draw the attention of boys and men (would, as my assistant principal had said, "distract other children"). I grew up in a conservative Christian household with traditional views on modesty and purity. While I bristled at the dress code, part of me realized just how dangerous it was to use women's dress to keep men accountable for their thoughts and actions and how unfair it was to place this burden solely on women. Women are asked to hide their bodies and dress modestly because a narrative exists that men can't control themselves mentally and physically. But when you place the onus on women, you unwittingly assign blame. If men have such a difficult time with self-control, why don't we teach them how to control themselves instead of focusing on the length of a woman's skirt? After all, the Bible says that if a man's eye causes him to lust, he should pluck out that eye—it's not a problem with the dress he's looking at, it's a self-control problem.

Now, I know that *modesty* is a relative term; it used to be immodest for women to show their ankles because men might become distracted if they caught a glimpse. It used to be scandalous for women to wear pants. Up until 1937, men were fined and arrested if they went topless at the beach! The definition of modesty is ever changing, but one thing remains the same—people dictate what is and isn't modest. We like to pin our own made-up or culturally shaped theology on God, but God made us naked and unashamed. Don't show your ankles, women can't wear pants, men can't be topless—these were never God's rules; they were society's. And people are still constructing rules for others based on their own personal convictions.

This became abundantly clear to me when I was thirteen and one of my aunts asked to speak with me privately. I was visiting her house, and my cousins were playing outside in the backyard. We sat in her living room surrounded by handmade quilts and natural wood furniture, only one cushion separating us on the couch.

I was nervous. I didn't know what she wanted to talk to me about, but I had a feeling in the pit of my stomach that it wasn't going to be positive. I was wearing a pair of jeans, a white T-shirt, and a hot-pink baby-doll dress. I was covered from chest to toe, but the bustline was fitted and accentuated my figure. I thought I looked cute and appropriate. (I always paid more mind to my dress when I visited this particular set of relatives. My mom is also one of seven children and has a large, expansive family. Some of my relatives make my parents' brand of conservatism look like socialism.)

My aunt stammered nervously; it was clear she wasn't entirely sure where to begin. "This is a little bit awkward," she said softly, "but, as a sister in Christ and your aunt, I just wanted to have a word with you about the way that you dress."

My heart sank into the depths of my already unsettled stomach. *Here we go again.* This was a topic that two of my aunts were always on my case about. Even after my parents told them they were not allowed to discuss clothing choices with me, they still made comments to me behind my parents' backs and out of their earshot.

"I've noticed the way that your cousins have been looking

at you recently," my aunt continued, "and I don't think you want them looking at you in that way. It's your responsibility to ensure you're leading them in the path of righteousness. The Bible instructs us that we are to be in this world but not of it. It urges us not to lead one another into temptation, and I would just ask that when you visit our home, you wear a sweater or a long skirt."

Once, on a family vacation when I was fifteen, another one of my aunts saw my thong peek above the waist of my pants when I bent over to get something. She made a big deal about how it wasn't appropriate for me to wear that type of underwear and told me that if she saw it again, she was going to "pull it." I didn't pay much attention at the time, but later in the day, as I sat next to one of my cousins building ginger-bread houses, she viciously pulled my underwear up so hard that my bottom came off the chair.

"Ow!" I exclaimed, tears flooding my eyes.

"I told you if I saw it, I was going to pull it," she replied with a shrug.

Sometimes I wonder how they would have treated me if I'd grown up with a different body—would a baby-doll dress over a T-shirt and jeans or a pair of underwear peeking out from my pants be as offensive? I'll never know.

These family members took modest dress seriously; for religious and other reasons, they opted to wear long skirts, long-sleeved, loose-fitting shirts, and heavy sweaters. And they instructed their girls to dress the same way. I, however, have always believed that people should wear whatever makes them feel best. I would never assume it was my re-sponsibility to instruct others on what they should wear.

Even though I view things differently from my aunts, I still love them fiercely. I also know that because of the way they were raised and their belief systems, they *thought* they were showing me love by correcting my dress. What they were actually doing was casually inflicting harm in the name of righteousness.

Even as a teenager, I understood that the issue wasn't me. It was a problem of misplaced resentment and blame with a little bit of nonbiblical church doctrine thrown in. I knew that arguing my case wouldn't end anywhere productive, and I valued the relationship too much to let it dissolve, so I respected my aunt's wishes. From that point on, when I visited, I wore a special sweater that I'd found in the men's department at Kohl's. It was hunter green with one big black stripe across the chest. It was big and bulky and kind of made me look like a square, but my aunt lit up with pride when she saw me in it. She would praise me: "My favorite sweater!" And it made me feel good to make her feel comfortable.

But in trying to keep the peace, I sacrificed something of myself. I've thought a lot about these memories over the years. At the time, I shrugged these incidents off as no big deal. I thought dressing a certain way to please them was a form of honoring and respecting their wishes. But when I look back, I can see that these interactions left me with deep, invisible wounds. I felt like they were really saying I wasn't welcome or allowed to be my true self around them, that my true self was a stumbling block on their path toward righteousness. It was another stone thrown at the body God had gifted me, a body that they, in the name of God, deemed too dangerous for me to fully inhabit.

6

Gut Feelings

Dear Body,
   Your intuition has never led us astray, but I
didn't always have the capacity to trust it. You came
equipped with an incredible sense for when things
were right, wrong, or just off. The older I get, the
more I realize that the feelings you give me in the pit
of my gut, soul, and spirit are there to protect me. I
am grateful that, despite the many times I've ignored
these signs, you persist and send them to me anyway.
I'm learning to listen.

When I was thirteen, my parents took me to a very special
dinner at the Pomona Valley Mining Company in Southern
California, a restaurant in a renovated old mine on top of
a hill with spectacular views of the city below. As dusk fell,
we sat together, just the three of us, surrounded by floor-to-
ceiling windows offering stunning views of the mountains
and the town twinkling with light. The sounds of tinkling

glass and silverware scraping on plates mingled with swirls of soft music and the rich, savory scent of roast chicken. The wooden table was immaculate, draped with a starched white tablecloth, a candle flickering in its center.

After the waiter took our orders, my mom looked at my dad; he gave her a nod. She reached into her purse, pulled out a small white box, and slid it my way. I opened it gingerly, and the candlelight caught the gemstones glittering inside. It was a white-gold ring with a blue zircon—my birthstone—in the middle. Down the sides were engraved crosses and pavé diamonds. I knew immediately what it was: a purity ring. And I was so grateful; I'd been reading literature on taking a purity pledge for months and it was something that meant a lot to me.

My mom pulled out a certificate and a pen.

"Brit, this is something we want you to sign, a promise to the Lord," my dad said with a smile. "We know you've expected it to come, and today's the day. We're so proud of you and we hope this encourages you to stay strong in your faith and commitment to save yourself for your husband."

As I scrawled my signature (which felt like the *coolest* thing to a new teen), my mom placed her hand on my dad's back.

They were so proud.

I put the pen down, turned the box to face me, and pulled out the ring. I placed it on my left ring finger, then turned my hand to show them. My dad pulled out his digital camera and snapped a photo of me smiling broadly, showing off my purity ring as if I'd just gotten engaged. And that huge smile on my face wasn't faked in any way. I loved that ring and everything it represented. I wasn't just trying to please my parents—I wanted to please the Lord.

As the waiter placed my Caesar salad with big, buttery croutons in front of me, I gazed out the window. Even then,

I knew that sex could be a way to get you to open up your heart before it was ready. Among my friends, virginity was a popular topic of conversation. *Are you one? Do you want to be?* And I knew that girls who weren't virgins were looked at differently from boys who weren't. I wasn't really concerned with anyone else's choices; I just knew that I believed sex was for marriage and that in order to honor God and my future husband, I wanted to wait.

For me, the highlight of every summer was spending a week with my grandma Sharon. My sister and I would often go visit her in her two-story home with palm trees decorating the yard. We had our own room, and we would stay up all night talking about life, family drama, and boys; take walks in the summer sun; enjoy the pool in her gated community; and, of course, go shopping—no expense was spared. I also had several second cousins who lived near her; they were older and seemed *so* much cooler than I was.

During family gatherings, it was normal for the kids to go off by themselves while the adults hung out together, enjoying bonding time without having to police the kids. With the steady sound of grown-up chatter and laughter as a backdrop, we kids would run loose, play silly games, and sometimes retreat to the back porch or the upstairs loft. One of my distant family members, Trey, always led the lot of us.

He was really handsome—tall, with a cool, effortless ease about him. He was four years older than I was, and we didn't see each other a lot, but when we did, I wanted him to think I was cool, someone fun to hang out with.

One night when I was thirteen and he was seventeen, all the kids were hanging out together on Grandma Sharon's back porch, and he looked over at me and said, "You know, one time my mom dated one of her cousins and it was actually really not that bad."

A lump formed in my throat. I didn't say anything; I offered an uncomfortable laugh in response.

"Come sit on my lap," he said, his lips curling into a crooked smile.

I wanted to say no, yet something held me back. Yes, he was four years older than me and he was *my relative*. But I really wanted him to like me—not *like me*-like me, but approve of me, acknowledge me. I also didn't want to hurt his feelings. I was taught to be nice, and in that moment, the nice thing to do seemed to be not insulting him. *Who is this hurting, really?* I thought.

I stood up from the couch and made my way over to him. He pulled me onto his lap. He nuzzled my neck. I could smell his Axe body spray, which made me feel a little sick, but I sat there anyway, stiff as a board, my smile frozen in place as he put his arms around my waist.

As I suppressed the feelings of discomfort, the agony of being held when I wanted to run, it dawned on me: This behavior—this compliance—*was* hurting someone.

It was hurting me.

Yet I brushed that feeling aside, shoved it down, and wrote it off as an overreaction.

A couple of summers later, my sister and I were visiting my grandma, and we were bored because she was working during the day. My grandmother called Trey and asked him to take me and my sister to the pool. She asked him to bring two of our other female relatives along, knowing that my dad wouldn't want us solo at the pool with a boy, relative or not.

My stomach flipped as I remembered the discomfort I'd felt the last time we'd hung out, but I was still excited to get out of the house and hang with some older kids. My sister and I packed up our things and got into our swimsuits.

When he arrived, all three of us walked to the pool. I was expecting to see our other relatives there, but they never joined us.

He hadn't invited them.

We walked through the pool gate, tossed our stuff onto the beige lawn chairs, and slid into the pool. We played around, splashing and laughing—it felt good to get a break from the strong California heat.

Soon, four of his friends from school showed up on bikes—all older, eighteen- and nineteen-year-olds. They greeted Trey with fist bumps and high fives, then waved at my sister and me. Trey jumped out of the pool, and he and his friends headed to the hot tub, leaving my sister and me alone. We kept swimming and chatting, though I was painfully aware that I had not been invited to hang out with them. I was fifteen, after all, and my sister was eleven; I wanted to be seen as a peer, not put in the same category as my sister, who I viewed as a little kid.

Not long after, one of the boys yelled, "Brittany, come here, we want to ask you a question."

I got out of the pool, feeling incredibly self-conscious and exposed as I walked toward them in my bathing suit, especially since I'd been told that bathing suits weren't particularly flattering on me. I awkwardly held my hands over my body, placing them strategically to cover my rolls, and I sucked my stomach in.

When I got to the edge of the tub, I looked around at the faces of the older guys. Two of them were pretty meh; one was super-cute. I stood there hugging my body until the guy who'd called me over said, "Get in here, we want to talk to you."

I came closer, but I stayed on the step and dangled my feet in the hot water.

"So," the good-looking guy asked, "do you think I'm cute?"

"Yeah, I think you're cute," I responded with a stifled laugh, my arms still wrapped around my midsection.

"Okay. But do you think I'm *really* cute?"

"Yeah," I said quietly. I expelled a huff of air, my eyes darting to the side, cheeks hot with embarrassment.

"Well," he said, wading toward me, "why don't you come over here and sit with me, then?"

Before I could say anything, he grabbed me off the step and pulled me onto his lap. That's when it hit me, like the sixth sense that hits a gazelle in the wild as she hears a branch break nearby: *I'm in danger.*

As he held me tightly, pressing my bottom against his lap, my eyes scanned the pool area. I was in the hot tub, surrounded by guys all much bigger and stronger than I was, with no way out and no adults around. There was no one else in the pool enclosure except for my eleven-year-old sister and some lady tanning way off in the corner with headphones on. I felt helpless and alone, isolated in my own fear. My mind raced as I tried to come up with ways to escape.

Even in that panicked state, I was still that nice girl who didn't want to embarrass herself in front of my relative's friends. I couldn't get up and say, *No, I don't want you touching me this way,* and run away. Even in the midst of my extreme discomfort and confusion, I was still somehow more concerned with not making *him* feel bad or rejected than with my own personal comfort or safety.

I tried to shake the fear, to relax into the situation. The

guys were talking, laughing, joking around. I pleaded with my brain to look at the situation differently. *I'm okay, this is just what cool girls do; they hang out with guys like this. They'll continue to talk, forget I'm here, and I'll casually leave in a few minutes.*

Finally, I said, "I think I'm going to go back in the pool. I need to check on my sister."

The boy said, "No, no, I want you to stay here." He hugged my body firmly so I couldn't move.

Again, I said, "I think I need to go check on my sister because she's by herself over there and she's only eleven."

He said, "No, I really think you should stay here," then started laughing.

Before I knew it, he had lifted me off his lap and was passing me to one of the other guys in the hot tub. That guy pulled me onto his lap and roughly grabbed my breasts. I was mortified and shocked out of my politeness.

With more courage and authority in my voice, I said, quietly but firmly, "I really want to get out now. I really want to go see my sister. Please get your hands off me."

He released my chest. I felt myself relax a bit; this was almost over. I was moving away from him—the edge of the tub was within reach. Then, just as I went to grab the lip of the tub, he lifted me and passed me to my relative.

In an instant, Trey had his hand down my top. My heart was racing; everything in my body shouted, *Get out now!* But I didn't fight or shout; I continued to sit quietly. I felt frozen. My silence was my concession but not my permission. I thought about God. I thought about how I'd betrayed Him by welcoming this. What had I expected when I got into a hot tub with five older guys? I was so stupid.

I enabled this.

They took turns passing me around, touching my body. One guy stuck his hand down my bathing-suit bottom, and another guy put his hand down my top. They finally passed me back to the original guy who'd called me over, and he started kissing my neck. That's when I physically pushed him away and said, "I really have to check on my sister."

I got out of the hot tub and ran to my sister, who was still floating there in her watermelon bathing suit, albeit a bit annoyed. She had a real sore spot about being left out. She always felt like she was in my shadow and resented that I was allowed to do things that she wasn't. I sank down next to her, wrapped my arms around myself, and told her what had happened. When I finished the story, she looked me in the eye, water dripping off her soaking hair, and said, "Well, yeah, 'cause that's what you wanted. You went over there to hang out with all of those guys. What did you think was going to happen?"

Immediately, shame covered me like someone had poured molten lava over my head—I evaporated into it. I'd thought it first; I'd been quick to blame myself, but to have someone confirm that blame solidified my distorted narrative about what had happened.

I'd asked for this.

I'd walked over to the hot tub on my own, wearing a bathing suit, which was basically underwear. I got into the hot tub. As they touched me, I didn't punch; I didn't bite, kick, or scratch. I was compliant. I let it happen.

Soon, we went back to Grandma Sharon's house. When I walked through the door, still wet from the pool, the air-conditioning felt frigid against my skin. I went to the bathroom, hung my wet towel up to dry, and leaned against the wall. I closed my eyes and used all the energy I hadn't been able to muster in the hot tub to push the memories out of my head. I kicked and shoved, scratched, bit, and fought with every detail until only a shadow of the memory remained. Then I looked down at my hand, my purity ring sparkling in the light from the bathroom window. I wondered if I should take it off.

7

Love

Dear Body,
    One of the most beautiful things about you
is your potential for love and intimacy. As we've
grown together, I have tried to share you only with
people who will treat you with dignity, reverence,
respect, and tenderness. I haven't always succeeded,
but I look back on my first taste of love and know
that I wouldn't be who I am today without those
experiences, and I thank you for it.

I grew up believing that I would meet the man who would become my husband in high school and we'd begin building a family in our late teens or early twenties.

My parents met when my mom was fourteen and my dad was seventeen, and many of my aunts, uncles, and cousins married young too. My favorite movies reinforced this "fall in love during high school" notion—*She's All That, Ten Things I Hate About You,* and *Clueless.* The adults I spent the most time with had all gotten married as teenagers; even the Bible seemed to push for young marriage, with verses like "It is better to marry than to burn with passion" (1 Corinthians 7:9). Have you ever met a teenager? Passionate, hormonal beings.

I was told to pray for my future husband, to consider the qualities I wanted him to have. I wrote him letters and love songs and read books priming me for his arrival and our subsequent marriage. Though I was encouraged to be on the lookout, I was not allowed to date. I was coaxed to find "the one" but told stories of good Christian couples who saved their first kiss for marriage. Finding "the one" seemed an arduous task in and of itself, but with the added restrictions that I was not allowed to date or get physical with boys, well, needless to say, no one was beating down my door.

I'd had a short relationship and awkward first kiss with a boy named Dean—a fix-up that was, believe it or not, partially arranged by my mother after she spotted him at a football game!—but I had yet to fall in love.

When I started working at Mimi's, that changed. I quickly made friends with everyone on staff, including a really tall, model-esque server who became my crush. His name was Chris, and I fell hard and fast for his flirtatious ways and ocean-blue eyes. He'd blare George Strait from the speakers of his old red Ford pickup and he smelled like California sunshine. There was this exquisite tension that just kept building, building, building toward . . . something. It was like the grown-up version of the boy who pulls your pigtails on the playground. I never knew if I should chase after him or go crying to my mother.

We were drawn to each other like magnets. I'd never felt anything like that with another person before. I wanted to be near him all the time, and when I wasn't near him, I was thinking about him.

One day, about a month after I started working at Mimi's, we were both sitting in the break room. I had already finished folding all of my silverware into napkins and he was still working on his, so I grabbed a pile of napkins and started to fold alongside him without saying a word.

Out of the corner of my eye, I saw him smile as he said, "Hey, that's my silverware."

"It's not going to fold itself," I said. I continued to fold and place each finished set on top of the others.

"I have it on good authority that I'm the fastest folder 'round these parts," he said with a slight Texas twang.

"Mmm, you don't say?" I murmured. "Have you started yet or am I just supposed to fold this whole bin for you?" I grinned, feeling clever.

"I like when you flirt," he said. "You do this cute little thing with your mouth—"

"Oh, I wasn't flirting," I denied.

He smiled. "Let's be real. When are we going to admit what's really been going on here?"

"Oh," I said, turning to face him, arms crossed over my chest, "and what, pray tell, has been going on here?"

He grinned. "You already belong to me."

Disarmed, I laughed. "I do?"

He nodded and looked at me with so much certainty. "You do."

Dropping the playful banter for a moment, I whispered, "You're gonna be trouble."

"Is that what this is?" he asked.

"Yes," I said with just as much certainty.

It got to the point where neither of us could deny our feelings for each other. One day my friend KellyAnne, another server from Mimi's, invited me to the mall after work to see a movie. I dreaded asking my parents—I'd never been allowed to go anywhere without either them or the supervision of a friend's mom or dad—but I did, and I was shocked when my mom actually said yes. She went over the rules: Straight there and straight back. No boys. No strangers. No boys. Keep the cell phone on. No boys. No R-rated movies. No boys ... You get the picture.

KellyAnne and I were sitting at the Starbucks in the new outdoor mall in town talking about work and boys when all of a sudden Chris came walking in with another guy from work. It was like I'd summoned him with my thoughts. I must have looked as surprised as I felt because KellyAnne just giggled as she pulled me toward him. Unbeknownst to me, KellyAnne and Chris had set this whole thing up. He knew I wasn't allowed to go out with boys, but he wanted to see me outside of work and away from my house.

I was completely convinced my parents were going to show up to check on me. I had to text them what movie we were seeing, what the theater number was, how long the movie was, when it started, when it was supposed to end, and what Starbucks I was going to beforehand. Chris knew I was nervous, so he said, "Since this was just a chance meeting, how could they get mad at you?"

I raised my eyebrows and responded, "Oh, trust me, they would get mad."

Because I was my parents' oldest child, I was their guinea pig. They were strict because they wanted to do it right. But, boy, were they *strict*. As an adult, I know that I'm better for it, but as a kid, I felt suffocated sometimes.

This wasn't just my first date; it was the first time I had ever broken their rules. I was just not that kind of kid. I am still not that kind of person; I am a rule follower. I toe the line. And if I do anything that crosses that line, I usually tell on myself because the guilt eats me alive.

But for that one night, I just wanted Chris to be my secret, my special thing.

Falling in love with Chris wasn't something I ever had to think about—it just was. Every. Single. Moment. *Was.* Every second with him felt like floating and I would think, *This is what it's all about. All the songs, all the movies, every line in every book, every poem, every painting.* The world was brighter and more vivid than ever before and I was happy. Blissfully, completely happy.

8

Touch

Dear Body,
   It can be difficult to regain a level of comfort with
physical touch with others when so great a trespass is
made against you. It may feel easier to withdraw from
affection than to open yourself up to the possibility
of being hurt again. Navigating and acknowledging
the fact that we were taken advantage of left us wiser,
though wary. In love, we were fortunate enough to
walk with those who desired to heal us instead of
harm us further.

I've always had a certain level of discomfort with physical
touch. From the time that I was a young kid, I found greeting
others with hugs hello or kissing people goodbye felt awkward and uncomfortable. So I was surprised at how comfortable I was with Chris's affection from the very start. Not only
was I okay with him touching me, I *wanted* to be touched by
him, which was an entirely new feeling for me.

One evening not long into our relationship, after a pretty intense make-out session, we sat on my front porch, still breathing heavily, and I mustered up the courage to ask how many girls he'd kissed like that. The number was lower than I'd expected.

"What about . . . other stuff?" I asked nonchalantly, looking down at my hands.

"Other stuff?" he said.

"Yeah, you know. Like, sex stuff." I tried to sound casual as I picked at the chipped purple polish on my nails.

"Are you asking me if I'm a virgin?" He smiled and pulled my feet into his lap.

I looked at him. "Yeah," I said, not at all shyly.

"I am." His reply was soft as he focused on massaging my legs. "I've done other stuff, but not that, not yet."

"You know my history." I pulled my legs away from him and hugged them against my chest. "I kissed Dean, then you . . . and . . ." I hesitated, then added quickly but quietly, "There was something that happened last summer with a group of boys, but I didn't really want that to happen."

He was quiet for a long moment before he said, "You don't have to tell me, but if you would like to tell me, I would like to listen."

I took a breath and told him about what happened the summer before in the hot tub. I told him everything—about my relative's flirty behavior, about wanting to protect my relationship with him, about being afraid to speak up because I didn't want to be mean. I told him about that day, how I was flattered to be asked to hang out, then how it all changed so quickly. "I made a really dumb decision, putting myself in that situation, and I'm sorry. I don't know if that classifies me as a nonvirgin now."

I glanced over at Chris. His face was contorted in a way

I'd never seen before. He looked horrified. "Oh," he said softly. "Oh, love, please don't apologize. Brittany, that wasn't just a kiss or something consensual and small that happened with an ex. That was sexual molestation. You were molested by those guys."

"What does that mean?" I asked, embarrassed that I didn't know.

"It's when someone touches you in an unwanted way without your consent or permission." He looked so sad. "Oh, man, Brit, I'm so sorry that happened to you." He took my hand in his and gave it a light squeeze.

"Wait," I said, still not quite grasping the magnitude of what I was being told. "I don't understand. I got into the hot tub. That was my choice."

"Just because you exist doesn't give anyone permission to lay hands on you. You didn't make any mistakes at all, not one, other than thinking this was in any way your fault. Those boys should be arrested; they could do this to some other girl, if they haven't already."

Chris encouraged me to tell my parents about what had happened. I was reluctant because I knew that they'd be upset, and I didn't want to get anyone in trouble. Looking back, I can see how the way I was conditioned to handle abuse colored my interaction with those boys. I was a peacekeeper, a parent pleaser turned people pleaser. It was easy for me to ignore my feelings of discomfort, hurt, or even pain so that my abuser didn't have to feel the weight of them. It wasn't even something I had to think about; prioritizing their feelings was automatic.

Over the years, I've thought a lot about why victims feel protective of their abusers. They struggle with the fear of conflict or the shame from coerced consent given under duress. When certain types of people hear a terrible story about a woman who was molested or raped, they'll ask, "What was she wearing?" or "Why was she there in the first place?" The same questions I had asked myself after my own sexual molestation. Those questions shift the blame from the abuser to the victim. As Chris said to me that night, your existence isn't an excuse for someone to mistreat or abuse you.

With Chris sitting on the other side of the door, I told my parents what had happened. My dad's eyes filled with tears, and my mom cried. I knew that they were sorry that I'd experienced something they were so desperate to protect me from. We all felt responsible in part for what happened, but the truth is that the blame rests solely on those boys.

Talking about the assault made a tangible difference in my life. I felt lighter, happier, and free from the burden of self-deprecating thoughts. My parents advocated on my behalf, even though it became a tangled mess of "he said, she said." Despite this, I was finally able to move on from that moment and let it go. I can only hope that those who have the courage to share their sexual assault or trauma are met with the same understanding, love, compassion, and reason that I was.

9

Moving

Dear Body,
   I always felt like we needed someone to save
us. Living at home felt like walking on eggshells;
we never knew when the floor was going to go out
from under us. Chris was like a buoy in the midst
of a storm. A safe place to find rest, someone who I
knew truly, unequivocally loved us. But I've learned
that someone loving you doesn't necessarily mean
he's your savior, as much as you might want or need
him to be. I looked to the wrong things to rescue
us, unintentionally ignoring that the power resided
within us all along. Thank you for encapsulating all of
my greatest triumphs and most terrible heartbreaks.

The year before I met Chris, my parents started talking about
relocating to Texas. Homes were more affordable there, and
Aunt Kim and Uncle Daniel had paved the way by moving
there first.

After Chris and I had been dating for a little over a month, my parents announced they were planning a family road trip to visit my aunt and uncle in Texas. Chris told me he couldn't shake the feeling that he was going to lose me if we moved. I could sense his inner struggle—should he try to get closer to me because I might be leaving or should he pull away because it had the potential to get messy?

The night before we left, he told me he was in love with me. He gave me a stack of essays and letters he'd written trying to articulate his feelings for me and telling me he was worried because they were so strong and it was so fast and we were so young. In the last letter, he shared his fears and his hope that I might love him too. He was scared I wouldn't say it back or that I was going to move to Texas and that would be it; we'd end before we really had a chance to get started. I was the first person he'd ever said "I love you" to outside of his mom and grandparents.

I kissed him deeply and snuggled up closer to him. We were parked under the streetlights in his old red truck. I confessed that I'd loved him from the moment I met him and that nothing would ever take that away. On the twenty-four-hour car ride to North Texas, I reread his letters at least a hundred times. And after we arrived, I spent most of my time telling Aunt Kim stories about my new friends, work, and Chris; the conversation always seemed to find its way back to him. My parents had no intention of looking for a new home on that trip, but they took to the wide-open spaces and wanted to come back to stay.

Part of me was excited. I'm a Sagittarius, so I love adventure, getting swept away in the tidal wave of destiny, subject and slave to the winds of change. The idea of starting anew is very appealing. I've always preferred wings over roots.

But I didn't want to leave Chris. We spoke several times

a day throughout that week. He'd made me a book of songs and a mix CD to take with me, including tracks like "Ain't No Mountain High Enough," "Faithfully," and the song he said he could have written for me himself, our song, "Shameless." He had carefully typed the lyrics for every song in a scrapbook and included a paragraph on what the song lyrics meant to him, what they meant for us, and the promises that he was making to me because of them. On the final page of the book, he'd written, *And if you haven't figured it out by now, there's no way that I'm letting you get away from me. If you move to Texas, I'm going with you.*

At the time, I believed that meant I could have both a new adventure in a new city and Chris. I was confident that we were strong enough to figure it all out. Isn't love supposed to conquer all?

Things moved fast after that trip. It wasn't long before my parents found a house in Texas and my mom got a job there, and our house in California sold in record time. This far-fetched dream was quickly becoming a reality, and I was desperate not to lose Chris. My parents had an extra room in the new house, and they offered to let him rent it until we got married.

One night, Chris picked me up after his shift at work to take me to dinner with his extended family. We were instructed by my parents to go straight to the restaurant and come right back. This was the first time my parents were allowing us to drive somewhere in the car alone together without a sibling chaperone and they didn't want any funny business. When I got in his truck, Chris said, "I have to make a quick stop at my place first to change and then we'll be on our way." I nodded and we listened to Keith Urban and chitchatted during the fifteen-minute drive.

When we got to his place, I realized I had to pee. I knew my parents wouldn't want us in his house alone together, but exceptions to the rules had to be made.

His pickup came to a stop inside his garage. It was the first time I'd ever been there. "Can I use your restroom?" I asked hesitantly.

"Of course!" he said. "I'm going to go upstairs and change, be back down in a sec." We went in, and he left me in the kitchen, pulling his white button-down out of his pants as he went. I made my way into the small downstairs bathroom of their town house and unzipped my skirt to pee. When I stood back up and tried to zip my skirt, the pesky zipper jumped the track. After I'd spent many minutes struggling, beads of sweat beginning to form on my face, Chris tentatively knocked on the door.

I recruited him to the mission, but once he realized he couldn't fix the zipper, he told me that we'd have to go back to my house so I could change, and he'd call his mom to tell her we were going to be a bit late. I was upset about that. There are few things worse to me than being late.

He told me my parents were going to laugh, that they would think it was funny—we sure thought it was. We were still laughing about it when we walked back through the door of my house. When my parents saw me holding my skirt together, they exploded.

"He was trying to take it off you and he ripped your skirt, didn't he?" my mother accused.

"No, that isn't what happened," I replied calmly.

"Oh, come on. Just tell us the truth," my dad said, his jaw clenched.

Their interrogation went on for ten minutes, making us even *later* for the family dinner. We were both insulted that they wouldn't believe us, but I was used to the way they jumped to conclusions. Chris wasn't—he said he'd never been treated like that by anybody in his life.

He went into dinner spitting mad and I was humiliated, worrying, *Is he going to stop loving me now?* But dinner went well; everyone was still waiting to be seated when we arrived, and after Chris quickly vented to his mom, the tension fell out of his shoulders, and the night went just fine.

That type of interaction came to define his relationship with my parents. They didn't trust us, and they *really* didn't trust him. They didn't believe anything that we, as a unit, said, even though we'd never given them any reason to doubt us.

When it was finally time to move, we drove to Texas in a three-car caravan. My mom drove a gigantic U-Haul, Dad drove a separate truck, towing a car, and Chris and I drove my dad's Excursion, another massive vehicle, pulling a second car behind it. I was sixteen and had just gotten my driver's license. Chris and I switched back and forth on the twenty-four-hour trip from California to Texas. The plan was to drive all the way through without stopping.

At one point, we both found ourselves falling asleep at the wheel and knew we needed to pull over. Chris radioed my dad and said, "Hey, Danny, we are going to pull off up here. We need some rest." So we all pulled off the road. Once we were parked, my dad and my mom got out of their trucks and started yelling, "Get out of the car! Get out of the car!"

When we were out of the car, my dad stormed over to us until he was in Chris's face. He bellowed, "You're a little boy! You don't ever tell *me* when to pull over." He went on. "What are you guys, infants? You can't just make it through?" He was still within an inch of Chris's face.

My mom decided to chime in, raising her voice too. She

shouted things like "Unbelievable" and "I can't believe the disrespect" and "Do you not value our time?"

When we got back in the car, Chris said, "I have never been yelled at like that, not even when I was a child. Human beings don't talk to other human beings that way."

My mind was blown. "Wait, your parents have never yelled at you?"

He scoffed. "Not like that."

"But your mom, she's never raised her voice?"

"It wasn't just their tone, Brittany, it was how close your dad was to my face, the demeaning words he chose. Come on, you know that's not right."

"Well, yeah, but they're my parents. I can't change how they are."

He shook his head. "I don't know. Do they always talk to you like that?"

I looked down, my hands folded in my lap. "Not always. Just when they get angry." He was quiet for so long I could feel the space stretch out between us, sitting side by side in the front seat of my dad's SUV but as far from each other as stars in the sky. The inky black nothingness separating us in a way I hadn't felt since we met.

Finally, he spoke again. "They are wrong." I looked at him, surprised. "They are so wrong," he continued. "It doesn't matter if they're your parents. You can't treat people that way." He looked at me and tucked a piece of hair behind my ear. "I'm so sorry you've been treated like that. I wish I'd found you sooner."

Chris wasn't the first person to shed light on the dysfunction within my family, but he was the most important. When aunts, uncles, or grandparents made comments, I was always quick to come to my parents' defense: "You don't understand—my dad has his own past to reconcile." "Mom never felt seen or heard as a child, that's why she screams." I was stalwart in their defense because I understood that their behavior didn't come from a lack of love; it came out of the tragedies they'd experienced themselves. And though I hated that the worst words ever spoken to me had fallen angrily from my parents' lips and some of the worst abuse I'd ever suffered had come at their hands, I was filled with compassion because I knew it was their pain that was spilling over onto me and my siblings. I was angry, but I was also fiercely protective.

However, when Chris told me what they were doing was wrong, I didn't feel protective anymore and I didn't want to defend their behavior or make excuses. At that moment, the abuse I'd suffered stopped being about them and their trauma and started being about me.

When we arrived in Texas, it was obvious that things between Chris and me were off. I didn't know if it was the cross-country trip or the altercation with my parents or something about me that was bothering him. He'd retreat to the backyard to call his mom and converse in private, his smile stopping before it reached his eyes. I decided to give him space. There were a lot of big life changes happening; he had a reason to withdraw and reflect.

After an afternoon of collecting job applications and speaking with college counselors about Chris's need to transfer and my need to enroll, we retreated to the back bedroom to fill out forms. I couldn't help but notice that as I scribbled away, Chris was still.

"Why aren't you filling out your applications?" I asked quietly.

"I'm not filling out applications because I'm not going to stay," he replied.

Time stood still.

He continued, his eyes filling with tears. "I just really need to go back home and finish school. It's not because I don't love you and it's not because I don't want to be with you, because I do—"

"But you don't," I accused, my cheeks as wet as his.

"Oh, but I do." He crawled closer to me and cupped my face in his hands.

"No," I cried softly. "If you did, you wouldn't be able to leave me. Not here."

I shed a lot of tears before I finally saw that he was right: It was madness for him to stay. I was sixteen. He was nineteen. He needed to finish school, be with his family. I told myself, *If he comes back to me, and this ends up working out, then that's what was meant to happen. And if not, then we weren't meant to be together in the first place, and we're better off. But we can still be friends. We can still care about each other.*

Looking back, I realize that he was not only my boyfriend, he was my best friend—and my escape plan. He was supposed to save me. I would be turning seventeen in six months. We were going to get married, and I would never have to live with my parents again. I wasn't just losing my first love and the man I thought I was going to marry, I was losing my way out. No teenage boy should have to shoulder all of that, and I knew it.

I will never forget the day he left.

"Tell me you believe me," he pleaded. "Tell me that you believe I love you."

I nodded, eyes wet. "I believe you."

"Tell me you understand why . . ."

"I do."

Nothing existed but the two of us, mourning the future we

once planned, watching it slip away. "This can't be the last time I ever kiss you. I cannot bear to think that this is the last time I'll kiss you," he whispered against my lips.

But it was.

Today, I am married, and Chris is married—and not to each other. But I still don't feel like that was the last time I'll ever see him. Life has a way of bringing people back to you.

I can't shake the feeling that one day, I'll be at a grocery store or the mall or a coffee shop, and I'll turn around and see him standing there. He'll say something like "Hey, how's life?" I'll tell him about Brady and my amazing kids and how he was right, that I used to make myself smaller to make other people feel better, but I'd stopped doing that, and even though it all turned out so differently than I'd planned, it turned out better than I'd imagined. I'll tell him that I hope it turned out better for him too. I did love Chris; my inner younger self still loves Chris. We had something rare, something I will forever hold close to me. It was a shaping love, a challenging love, a love that helped me learn who I was outside of my family. It helped me step into my identity.

And while Chris was the right boyfriend for me while I was discovering my power, I'd eventually find the man who was right for me as I grew into my power, and it would feel like something else entirely.

10

Battle Cries

Dear Body,
    I often felt like you were at war with me, that you wanted to hurt me or defeat me. Now I realize you were never my enemy; what I thought were battle cries were cries for help. The pain, fatigue, sleeplessness— this was your way of saying I was hurting you, that you needed me to stop, and that only I could bring about a cease-fire.

I buried my post-breakup heartache in busyness and swallowed my loneliness with food. By now, I'd become a master at avoiding pain, and I prided myself on having thick, impenetrable skin. Did things not hurt me the way they did others or was I just very good at acting like they didn't? I didn't know. I marched onward, ignoring the gaping hole inside me that Chris had left.

    Life in Texas was different from life in California, partly because I was growing up. I had two full-time jobs, one of which was at Barnes & Noble. Convenience became not just a luxury, but a necessity. I carried extra clothes in the back of my car so I could manage a quick change between jobs. And because I was on the go nearly 24/7, all my meals came from a drive-through window.

I became fluent in dollar menus and lived off McDonald's, Taco Bell, and the Barnes & Noble Starbucks Café, where I got 50 percent off sandwiches, cheesecake, and coffee. Food was no different when I had a rare day at home. My parents dealt with the stress of feeding seven kids by removing the stress from the process entirely. They would buy gigantic packs of pizza rolls, bagel bites, corn dogs, chicken nuggets, French fries, fish sticks, and hot dogs from big-box stores. Our family would go through eight gallons of milk every five days, so whenever we shopped, we would have a cart just for the milk. They also loaded up on sugary cereals, like Cinnamon Toast Crunch, Fruity Pebbles, Cap'n Crunch, and Froot Loops. Our pantry was the stuff of children's birthday-party dreams.

In a typical day at home, we'd start off by eating one or two bowls each of cereal with 2 percent milk. We were always hungry, no matter what we ate; a lack of micronutrients, vitamins, minerals, and healthy macronutrients in our meals fueled this unending hunger. We were bottomless pits. For lunch, we typically ate something quick, like the bagel bites, pizza rolls, or corn dogs. For dinner, it was stuff that we could fix for ourselves, like hot dogs and French fries or bean and cheese burritos. We never ate vegetables—they were rarely available to us. We existed on processed foods that contained little to no nutrient density or nutritional value. It was all empty calories and highly processed filler foods.

As a result, my body's natural full signal had been disabled; despite eating food, I was not getting the nutrients I needed, so my body was starving. This incessant hunger led to constant overeating, a pattern spurred on by manufactured foods that are engineered to override the body's natural hunger cues.

By this point in my life, it was no secret that maintaining my weight was a true struggle. But creating lasting change by modifying my diet or behavior seemed impossible. How do you create a healthier eating pattern when everyone around you carries on with the old, easier, and in many ways more appealing patterns?

The way we ate was normal to me; our lifestyle was normal. Processed cereals, frozen meals, fast food—this was what people ate. It was all I knew. Eating vegetables, fruits, and grilled chicken was not normal; you ate that stuff only if you were on a diet. I don't think this was just the case in my family. In the United States, we've normalized eating junk and processed foods to the point that eating real food is considered going on a diet.

I was so enslaved to processed and sugar-filled foods that it was virtually impossible to maintain any kind of healthy eating regimen. I'd go through periods where I'd decide to try eating healthy. But without anyone modeling what that looked like, I had no idea what to do or where to begin. So I would cut up one of the only vegetables that we ever had in the fridge, iceberg lettuce. I would smother it in Kraft Thousand Island dressing—the first ingredient of which is high-fructose corn syrup—and I'd eat an entire sleeve of saltine crackers on the side. (I assumed they were healthy because that's what people ate when they were sick.) I'd rinse all of it down with a Sprite, which was clear, so I figured it was basically flavored water. Or with Country Time lemonade, which was just powdered lemons, right? I would purchase one-dollar Smart Ones meals at the grocery store or one-hundred-calorie cans of soup, not paying attention to the fact that these "food-like" products might have been low in calories, but they were also severely lacking in any actual nutritional value. All of this led to cycles of restriction and then bingeing when the hunger became too great. My intentions were good—I wanted to be healthy—but the execution was all wrong.

My life was a house of cards crafted precariously on a rickety old table, bound to collapse with one kiss of the wind. My hair began to fall out in handfuls; I gained fifty pounds in three months; the light rash that I always carried on my upper arms intensified and spread to other parts of my body. I wasn't sleeping; I couldn't. My body was screaming the words my mouth refused to utter.

My mom began to worry, so she took me to the doctor, and I was diagnosed with hypothyroidism. I saw an endocrinologist who told me that I was at high risk for thyroid cancer and that I would be on medication for the rest of my life. Side effects of having an underactive thyroid are rapid weight gain, inability to lose weight, chronic fatigue, hair loss, muscle weakness, cold intolerance, brittle nails, and irregular periods. I thought, *Finally, an explanation.* But what it really felt like was an excuse. I was excused and absolved of my actions toward my body because I had a disease, something medical, something that couldn't be helped. No one ever mentioned that dietary changes might improve things. I was simply given a prescription for Synthroid and instructed to come back in six weeks for more blood work.

I hadn't yet connected my food choices, my lack of sufficient water, sleep, and movement, and the emotions I was suppressing to the way my body seemed to be rebelling. I didn't realize that food and emotional trauma could have such a huge impact on your body's overall well-being, not just on your weight.

—

As it turns out, I wasn't that great an actress. To those who knew me, it was clear that I was struggling to keep myself together because I was afraid of what might happen if I let myself fall apart.

"Are you okay?" Aunt Kim asked one afternoon in her living room as I popped Wendy's French fries smothered in ketchup into my mouth between big spoonfuls of a Frosty. She squinted at me and looked hard as she said, "Like, *really* okay?"

I paused between bites, feeling a little heat flood my cheeks, before answering her. "Yeah, of course!" I said, infusing my words with perkiness. She looked like she didn't buy it, so I followed it up with "Why do you ask?" I was careful not to say *Why wouldn't I be?* because there were a lot of reasons why I wouldn't be, and I didn't really want to get into all of that.

She sighed. "You just haven't seemed quite like yourself lately is all." She set her cup of chai tea on the table next to her.

"What do you mean?" I gave her my full attention.

"You've stopped wearing makeup," she said. "Not that you need makeup, but I know that it's something you've always enjoyed. You wore pajamas to work today. When was the last time you washed your hair? I'm just worried. Ever since Chris left . . ." She let her words hang in the air.

I bit the inside of my cheek and thought, *I guess we are getting into all of that.*

Sometimes the best thing a good friend can do is bring you to your own attention. "I know," I said quietly. I took a deep breath, building up the courage to whisper the words my body had been screaming for months. "I'm just really sad," I confided. "And I don't know how to make myself un-sad. Every day I wake up and he's gone. He's just gone and I didn't get to choose that, and it doesn't seem fair that he would make me love him just to have to lose him." Tears slipped down my face and I was as powerless to stop them as I was to stop my whispered confession. "He took so much from me, and I am so afraid that I'm never going to get it back."

"Oh, baby," Aunt Kim said softly. She crossed the space between us and wrapped her arms around me in a big hug. That embrace, knowing she was there for me, made me feel better. It didn't make me hurt less—the sadness didn't disappear— but letting someone know that I was not okay made it all feel a little less heavy. I didn't have to carry this weight alone.

I weighed nearly two hundred pounds at that point, but I didn't really pay much attention to how much I'd gained until one day when my mom and I went shopping at Kohl's. I gathered armfuls of clothing from the juniors department and made my way back into the dressing room. I hated trying on clothes. It was a miserable, sweaty experience; the clothing seemed to delight in highlighting my flaws. It was like the clothes had a vendetta against me, and in some ways, I guess they did.

I struggled to pull on a pair of the largest size pants but kicked them off aggressively when I couldn't get them over my thighs. I got stuck in a top and began to panic as I flailed around, cursing the world, terrified I'd have to call 911 so someone could cut me out of it.

"It doesn't fit! None of it fits!" I exclaimed as I burst out of the dressing room, the shirt still caught around my head and arms, uncaring that I was flashing my bra to the shoppers around us. "Mom! Help me get out of this death trap!"

I was only seventeen, and I couldn't shop in the juniors department anymore. As a girl who'd once loved fashion and drama, dressing for the world that was my stage, I was disappointed to see that the XXL options I had to choose from were . . . let's just say *very* lacking. Did clothing manufacturers actually think that women with bigger bodies should only dress like grandmothers? Later, I would come to understand this stark contrast in clothing style and availability between straight and plus-size clothes as "fat bias," or the social stigma against obesity. This bias has caused disadvantages for overweight people, creating stereotypes and prejudices that affect everything from employee/employer relationships to medical care to clothing and even our daily interactions with one another.

Even though I struggled at times with the way my body had changed, I always valued myself. I always saw myself as somebody who had a lot to offer, someone filled with promise, potential, love. But over time, I shifted the way I chose to see myself. I began basing my value almost entirely on who I was on the inside, as I didn't much care for who I'd become on the outside.

You can't change your relationship with food until you change your relationship with your body. It would be years before I realized that I had to start treating my body the way I treated other people—with kindness, compassion, and respect. I would have been appalled to hear someone talk to one of my friends the way I spoke to my body. But you're fluent in what you practice, and my inner dialogue revolved around what I perceived were my worst traits and qualities. I had years of unspoken emotional needs, traumas still yet to be healed, and my real, lasting desire for change wouldn't come for a while yet.

But when it did, it came from a place of love rather than a place of hate. You can't hate yourself to happy or criticize your way to change. The catalyst came from loving my body so much that I wouldn't rest until I helped her heal.

11

Schooled

Dear Body,
   I've always admired how hard we try, and I am
grateful for our willingness to adapt and make the
best out of every situation. Never giving up or settling
for less than what we know we are capable of, always
reaching, reaching, reaching toward the stratosphere
and outward toward the galaxy of our potential.

Making friends had never been hard for me, and I assumed that finding friends in Texas would come just as naturally as it always had. Not long after my breakup with Chris, Aunt Kim encouraged me to check out the youth group at her new church, and I thought getting closer to God and forming new relationships might be just what I needed to pull me out of my gloom.

I showed up a little early that first Wednesday night, right before the meeting began. I sat down in the back row of the youth room and watched as people wandered in and mingled, grabbing slices of pizza and waving to friends as they walked through the door. I brought my brother Colin with me as a sort of shield so that I didn't feel alone, but I still felt awkward. We sat in silence, watching everyone laugh and have conversations, feeling like outsiders who didn't belong. We ended up leaving right after the meeting without having spoken to anyone.

Colin didn't want to go back to the group, but I did. I hadn't made any friends, but the band that was leading worship had been awesome, and the youth pastor gave a good sermon, so the next Wednesday I showed up again. This time I grabbed a slice of pizza but kept close to the wall, trying to strike a balance between "open to conversation" and "not too intrusive." But as the group leader dimmed the lights and asked people to take their seats, I had to admit to myself that making friends might be more difficult than I'd thought. I sat in the back row by myself again, feeling kind of down.

I spent months trying to break into the airtight cliques that had formed far before the group's inception. While I made little progress, I became friendly with the worship team, who were mostly guys. They invited me to their band practice after I told them I could sing and play piano. Then one Wednesday, I was handed a microphone and asked to sing some BGVs (background vocals). But during sound check, the head pastor popped his head in and said he wanted me to take the lead on one of the songs.

I was shocked, embarrassed, and ill prepared. Stage fright, performance anxiety—they had nothing on the pressure I felt when first asked to help usher people into the presence of the Lord. My head was a mess—*You're too young, you still have so much to learn about God yourself*—and the song's key was just slightly outside of my comfort range, but I sang out anyway. I was glad it scared me, because it made me do it humbly.

Getting involved in church worship marked a turning point in my life. It felt like I had found my purpose. I was able to use my musical gifts to point people back to the source of life, of joy, and of love, and in turn, I reconnected to the source and began to heal.

Don't get me wrong—my life wasn't suddenly devoid of issues. I was still lonely, I had no local friends, and I missed Chris, but there was a supernatural calmness within my spirit that told me if I kept trying to honor and pursue God, it would all turn out okay. There's a verse in 1 Corinthians 13: "When I was a child, I talked like a child, I thought like a child, I reasoned like a child. When I became a man, I put the ways of childhood behind me." When I was a child, I didn't have a relationship with God. I had a learned understanding of Him, but not an emotional revelation or connection to the source of who He actually is. This was apparent in many ways but in one way particularly: I had a bit of self-righteousness. I felt that because I was good, better at following the rules than others, that somehow made me holier.

My desire to please God was much like my desire to please my parents. I wanted to win favor, but not out of love—out of fear and obligation. I also liked how being a good Christian girl garnered me positive attention from adults and boys alike. At the time, I didn't realize that I was manipulating my morality and spirituality to gain approval and esteem. It was subconscious, maybe even a survival mechanism of sorts, but it was always there as an undertone.

I didn't just *think* that I was special; I believed it. There were things about me that set me apart. Loud, noisy things that easily drew attention, and I've never been one to shy away from the spotlight. My parents, along with my teachers, aunts, uncles, even boyfriends, all told me that I would do amazing things. While this wasn't inherently bad, sometimes it fed the superiority complex I was developing. I had to learn to temper my unwavering belief in myself with humility and modesty. My faith also needed refining and maturing.

Moving to Texas was a gift of sorts—not one that I wanted, but one that I desperately needed. Because the truth is, we are all incredibly unique and special, and the flip side of the coin is also true—we are all very much the same.

Before my heartbreak and before we moved to Texas, popularity had come easy to me. My dynamic personality coupled with my extroverted nature made making friends as easy as breathing for me. I was different—fun and flirty—and outspoken about everything. I didn't just dance to the beat of my own drum, I created a symphonic orchestra, and I loved that I was seen as an enigma. Or maybe I just loved to be seen.

I can't help but cringe as I write this, and it makes me hate my younger self a little. But this was where my head was when I was a teenager. Like many other teens, I had "the world revolves around me" syndrome. These days I'm pretty familiar with my personality flaws. I've often struggled with selfishness and have the tendency to be harsh or biting with my words because I am so uncensored and honest. Oh, and I always feel like I'm right . . . always. I am a Sagittarius sun and rising with a Gemini moon, a seven wing three on the Enneagram, and an ENFP Myers-Briggs personality type— these traits are hardwired, and I'm the first to admit that I'm a work in progress. But as a teen, I wasn't as self-aware.

After relocating to Texas, I felt completely lost in the crowd. Suddenly it seemed that many of the things I'd thought made me special were so common it was almost annoying. My big personality was dwarfed by the appeal of quiet, mysterious girls who didn't wear their emotions or opinions on their sleeves. I was loud and boisterous. A modest church mouse, I was not. I never really fit the mold, and being in Texas made that apparent.

I was also reckoning with this feeling of being surrounded by overwhelming sameness: It seemed that everyone had the same goals, aspirations, and thoughts on life. I missed the diversity of culture, religion, politics, and people in California and the way these differences constantly inspired me to learn more, be more, and do more. For the first time in my life, I began to compare myself to other girls. Everyone was so tall, blond, and athletic that after a while, I didn't just feel lost in the crowd, I felt like I didn't even belong in the crowd—something that I'd never experienced before.

Christian culture prides itself on being welcoming, yet I was finding it difficult to form friendships in the church. I began to wonder if my weight had something to do with it; after all, when I was a more socially acceptable size, making friends had never been an issue. But at seventeen, five feet two and three-quarters, and two hundred pounds, as much as I tried, I didn't seem to be anyone's first choice as a friend.

Luckily, something came along that changed all that. Once a year, my church youth group went to the Desperation Conference—a huge youth conference at New Life Church, a megachurch in Colorado Springs, Colorado. When I was eighteen, about a year and a half after I moved to Texas, I was eager to go. It was a weeklong adventure, filled with dynamic worship, amazing speakers, white-water rafting, ropes courses, laughter, and lots of junk food. My parents were skeptical about letting me attend, but after the head pastor outlined the numerous safety measures in place, and my parents realized I was able to pay my own way, they relented.

74

On the last day of the conference, I wandered the lobby of New Life with Carter, a friend of mine through the worship team. Together, we browsed the tables promoting schools, faith-based organizations, and mission trips. Out of the corner of my eye, I noticed a table for the School of Worship, an accredited program through King's Seminary, sponsored by New Life Church. Carter stopped in front of the table, picked up a flyer, and flipped it over in his hands. Then he handed it to me, saying, "The Lord told me that you should go to this."

I laughed. "Yeah, right."

"I'm serious." He smiled. "This fall, this is where you'll be— Colorado."

Immediately, a lump formed in my throat. The prospect of higher education had always terrified me. I wasn't even certain my parents would allow me to attend college.

The truth was, I had only finished seventh grade.

Let me back up. When we were living in California, we faced a number of challenges when it came to school. It's a very diverse state, and the income gap is massive. When I was in middle school, we moved to a house in a lower-income part of town so our housing would be more affordable but we'd still have access to a good school. All told, it was an okay school, but there was a wide disparity in how the students behaved—people either kept their heads down or were bullied mercilessly and harassed. There was gang activity, and we had metal detectors and cops on campus. It wasn't uncommon for guys to grab your breasts or your butt in the hallway. In seventh grade, I had rejected one of the more popular guys, so he started calling me "Twenty-Five-Cent" to imply I was a twenty-five-cent whore. All the boys in my class followed along. I lived with that nickname for an entire year.

That same year, my brother got into a fight with one of his classmates. The other boy started it and my brother was just defending himself, but our school had a zero-tolerance policy for fighting. It didn't matter who started it—anyone caught fighting was expelled and arrested with an automatic misdemeanor and court date. The only way to expunge the record was through community-service hours.

My parents were understandably upset and decided that our school district was no longer a safe place for us. They let us finish the school year, and the following September, they started homeschooling us.

That summer, my parents went to their first homeschool conference, and they got super-jazzed about the idea. They bought a computer-based curriculum and a couple of computers, and when summer ended, school was officially in session. I was excited too, at first, especially after the humiliating year I'd had in seventh grade. I was really devoted for the first couple of weeks; so was my dad. He would tell us to go do our work, then he would walk around and make sure that we were following along and understanding everything. But after a while, he stopped looking over our shoulders to see if we were completing our assignments. (In his defense, he was taking college courses online and working toward a master's degree himself.) So we all just . . . stopped. Our parents had given us everything that we needed to teach ourselves, but without any accountability or structure in place; we had no formal supervised schooling.

The saving grace for me was my passion for reading. I practically ate books for breakfast. *Gone with the Wind* was one of the first big books I read cover to cover. Then I read anything my mom and dad had in the house: Grisham, Koontz, King, Austen, Dickens, Fitzgerald. When I exhausted my parents' relatively limited collection, I started going to neighbors' houses and borrowing from theirs. That's where

I discovered my love for romance novels that left me with flushed cheeks and a racing heart.

My parents had more faith in the education system in Texas, so when we moved there, they made the decision to enroll us in public school again. They gave me the option of either "officially" graduating from homeschooling or beginning high school as a freshman, given my level of education. But two of my younger brothers were also enrolling as freshmen, and being held back three years did not at all appeal to me. Previously I'd been in GATE (gifted and talented education) classes; I could read at a twelfth-grade level when I was nine, and I was doing college algebra in fifth grade. At sixteen, I should have been a junior or a senior taking dual-credit college courses, not starting my freshman year. I felt robbed of an opportunity and the promise of what my life once held.

Not loving either option, I told my parents to officially graduate me. In the state of Texas, all you need to graduate from homeschool is your parents' say-so. They said so, my dad drew up a diploma and a transcript, and I enrolled in college. I tried to tell myself that I was lucky; few other sixteen-year-olds could brag that they'd already graduated high school. But I knew that I hadn't really done the work, and I resented my parents' pulling us out of an organized education system.

Looking at that flyer brought all of these emotions back. I'd envisioned that I would sail through college the same way I'd been able to sail through school, but those missing years symbolized a lot of loss—a loss of not just my education, but my friends and life back in California, my potential. College was something I no longer dared to consider. It was a dream of the past, a direction my life could have taken but didn't. I felt like that door was firmly closed. I was terrified of being exposed as a nineteen-year-old woman with a seventh-grade education. I imagined others seeing me like one of the Lost Boys from *Peter Pan*: dirty, wild, and ignorant. So when Carter gave me the pamphlet for the School of Worship, I stuffed it in my bag and decided the best course of action was to let my parents veto the idea. I was absolutely positive that they'd be against my leaving home and moving out of state.

Surprisingly, that's not what happened at all; my parents thought it was a great idea. There was only one explanation for this: What Carter said must have been true. This was where the Lord wanted me to be for the next year. I took their encouragement as partial confirmation and decided to apply. While the school got hundreds of applications every year, it admitted only forty students at a time. I knew my chances were minimal and told the Lord that if I was accepted, I would take it as final confirmation that I should attend seminary in Colorado.

Just a few weeks later, I received my acceptance letter. It was a strange feeling—I wanted to go, but I was afraid that I wouldn't be able to keep up. I also carried a large amount of unresolved and unspoken resentment toward my parents. I blamed them for a lot of things—not just my lack of formal education but also being overweight, having an autoimmune disorder, and losing Chris. I had all of these hard emotions that I didn't know what to do with, and it was easier to blame my problems on them because that absolved me of responsibility and allowed me to avoid taking action.

I held on to these resentments for a long time. Eventually and with a change in perspective, I was able to shift the way I viewed things. By acknowledging that I was hurt by these trespasses and determining not to let my parents continue to trespass, I transferred control of the situation from their behavior, which I couldn't control, to mine, something I could. I realized that my bitterness poisoned me more than it did them and that ultimately I didn't want to poison our relationship.

Now I love the fact that I wasn't formally educated. I think that it gives me a different perspective on the world, and I look back fondly on those years when I did nothing all day but daydream, write songs, and devour book after book. Non-schooling unintentionally encouraged my hunger for education and learning, whereas traditional school often felt more like a job and diminished it.

My parents certainly did not do things by the book, but was it wrong? I can't say that it was, especially knowing how well we all turned out. Two of my brothers own a demolition company with my dad, another brother is a paramedic, and my sister is an operations specialist at a very successful company. Releasing my resentment gave me the power to own my situation and make something grand out of it.

Without a doubt, Colorado was exactly where I was destined to go that year. It would just take me a bit of time to realize that.

12

Saved

Dear Body,
    I love our ability to grow physically and mentally.
Moving to Colorado was a life-changing experience;
it equipped us with the knowledge that we were
capable of so much more than we knew. Taking a
risk or a chance on ourselves is never a bad idea. Jim
Carrey once said that you can fail at what is safe and
comfortable or you can fail at what you love, so why
not take a risk on what you love?

At first, I doubted that Colorado was the right place for me.
After several months, I hadn't made any friends; I was spending so many hours working there just hadn't been time. I had
a rough start with my first housing situation, a rented room
in a creepy family home that was clearly not a fit, so I was
suddenly homeless. But my luck began to turn when a girl
in one of my classes, Rachel, heard about my situation and
spoke with her roommate about it. They offered to let me

move in with them. We would have to share a bedroom, she explained, but it would help them out, as they were struggling to make rent, and I could sleep on the couch or on her air mattress. I was a kid from a big family, so sharing a room was nothing new to me, and I immediately agreed.

Although living with Rachel and Janna was rough at first—they'd been best friends for years, and Janna felt a bit threatened by the relationship I'd built with Rachel—Janna eventually came around, and those girls made my school year. We ate half-price happy-hour appetizers at Applebee's together, nearly froze to death through a Colorado winter with no heat in our very crappy apartment, and worked bizarre odd jobs to pay the bills. We bonded over boys we were halfway in love with who didn't know we existed, fought over who should do the dishes and take out the trash, and got tattoos. They looked like me, they thought like me, they loved music like me—for the first time in years, I felt like I belonged.

It was the first experience in the adult world for all three of us, and we were doing it together. Suddenly, that world didn't seem so scary anymore. I liked not having to ask for permission to see a movie with a friend. I loved buying my own groceries. I had made a comfy little home with my roommates in a rundown old apartment building where I paid my share of the rent—one hundred and sixty dollars a month—and slept in the living room on an orange-and-brown-plaid love seat from the 1970s because the air mattress deflated and money was too tight to purchase another mattress for the bedroom. We didn't have heat or AC, we could hear our neighbors talking through the walls, I found used condoms in the parking lot, and I shared a bedroom, but it was all ours and for the first time in my life I felt empowered, knowing that I was completely capable of taking care of myself.

I made enough money to become independent from my

parents, and I had friends. Those lonely months in Texas when I couldn't seem to connect, even at church, seemed so far away. I thrived in Colorado, standing on my own two feet, paying my own bills, getting great grades—I'd been waiting my whole life for someone to rescue me, but my time in Colorado taught me that I could rescue myself.

Moving to Colorado ignited something within me and gifted me with new adventures, independence, and growth. I formed deep, lifelong friendships while learning about theology, apologetics, and the history of the religion I hold so dear. My faith expanded; my understanding grew; and I felt the evolutionary tug of growth on my heart and my mind. I fell in love with school again, and the knowledge that I was capable of doing challenging things was awakened within me, ushering in an entirely new stage of my life.

It was a one-year program, and as the year came to a close, I felt like a new person, one who was much more confident and much more independent. There was a burning desire in my heart to stay in Colorado; I was afraid I'd lose all of this progress if I went back home.

After I graduated, a friend invited me to rent one of the rooms in her house for three hundred dollars a month. I was waitressing at Applebee's and I'd grown to love the church community in Colorado Springs. I had an aunt and uncle who didn't live far away, so I even had a sense of family there. I decided I was going to stay and continue to explore life on my own in the beautiful mountain town.

I knew that my parents wouldn't love my decision to stay; I knew they missed me and were excited for me to move back home. But I hoped that they would support and respect my choice. My friend held my hand as I called my parents to tell them my decision. I was twenty; I expected them to be sad, but I didn't expect them to tell me no.

In that one call, the self-confidence I'd gained in Colorado began to falter. One moment I felt like I'd made a solid, rational decision and the next I was frustrated and questioning myself. My parents told me that they'd allowed me to go to Colorado only because I was in ministry school and under the umbrella of the church's protection. Now that I'd graduated and left the safety of the church behind, they reasoned that it was their responsibility to protect me again. They said that if I stayed in Colorado, I would willfully be choosing disobedience. They made it clear that, in their eyes, I would be making the choice to reject my father's protection.

I felt completely torn between the life I'd begun to build and the life that had been built for me. I wanted to stay in Colorado so badly, but I had been trained for twenty years to obey. I could see the tatters of my freedom slipping through my fingers, so I did what I always do when I feel helpless: I called Aunt Kim. She said that I was an adult and could choose to do whatever I liked, but she reminded me that you could never go wrong in choosing your family and she suggested I pray on it.

I learned a long time ago that if you pray about something more than you talk about it, the Holy Spirit will give you clear direction. Even if it's not the direction you were hoping for. I'd decided that I was going to live a life in which I surrendered to the Lord as much as I could. In our hearts, we plan our course, but the Lord establishes our steps (Proverbs 16:9). So instead of talking to anyone else about what to do, I prayed.

I wrestled with my decision as I placed it at the feet of the Lord. If I stayed in Colorado, it could mean the end of my relationship with my parents. If I went back home, it would be like signaling to my parents that they still had total control over my life. It would mean returning to a house of friction. I couldn't afford to live on my own in Texas—I didn't have any potential roommates or even a job. I would have to, at least for a time, become financially dependent on my parents again. It would undoubtedly blur the lines of the already fragile boundaries I'd begun to establish.

Trauma encourages you to shutter up your heart, but healing encourages openness and clear boundaries. The distance of that year had facilitated a healthier relationship between me and my parents. It made establishing boundaries easier because they didn't require daily reinforcement; there was less opportunity for friction. Absence didn't just make the heart grow fonder; it made our relationship healthier. I was utterly torn.

And then I felt a nudge.

My spirit said, *Go home.* As I continued to listen to my spirit, the message became clearer. *Don't do it for them. Don't do it out of obedience or honor or umbrellas of protection but because there is something unfinished at home.* Suddenly, I could feel it so strongly—a pull. Something was calling me back. Even though I worried about what it would be like to return to the dynamic of my family's home, I knew in my gut that I was supposed to return to Texas.

And so I went.

13

Walking in Faith

Dear Body,
   I value our ability to prioritize what is best over what we feel. Choosing to go back to Texas when I desperately wanted to build a new life in Colorado felt so difficult at the time. Taking that step was truly walking in faith. In retrospect, our whole life would have taken a different course if we hadn't gone back home.

Going back home was as easy as fitting a snake into a skin it had already shed. I was a changed person trying to play a role I had aged out of. Some might be comforted by and content to stay on the path of least resistance, but I felt trapped and confined by it. When I returned to North Texas, I enrolled in a community college, and I decided to change my major from biblical counseling to elementary education. If I worked hard, I would finish school within two years. I didn't want to take out student loans, so I went back to juggling three different jobs so I could pay my way as I went. Once I had a career, I could afford an apartment. Being a teacher would allow me to travel during breaks and I would have the summers to do with as I pleased. It seemed ideal.

I had realized I was more than capable of taking care of myself, and for the first time in my life, I wasn't looking for a boyfriend, and I wasn't making decisions based on the assumption that a husband and kids were right around the corner. I liked being single.

Even though I had changed, the world around me hadn't; my friends and family desperately wanted me to live life a certain way because they believed it was the best life a woman could have. There was still the push from friends and family: "Why aren't you dating?" "It's so sad that you don't have love in your life." "I already had three kids at your age." My inner truth was at constant war with what I had been taught to believe.

It was almost like they just wanted me to check boxes off a list. Get married—check! Have babies—check! And then what? Don't get me wrong, I wanted those things eventually. And yet I couldn't fully comprehend *why* I wanted them. Was it because they were what I'd been conditioned to want or because I actually desired them? I wasn't sure, but I did know that they weren't at the top of my priority list any longer. I was done waiting to plan trips to faraway places because it was something I wanted to save to do with my spouse. I had friends to share experiences with now. And I felt like the whole wide world was mine to explore.

Within a week of being back home, I was offered a position on staff at my home church. It was easy to slip back into that role; seamless, even. I don't even remember a discussion; it was just assumed that I'd go back to leading worship. It was what I'd gone to school for, after all. I began assisting the children's ministry director and the worship pastor while leading worship in children's ministry and co-leading church services on Sunday mornings and Saturday nights. It was going well and it was fulfilling work, but I missed feeling challenged the way I had in Colorado. Emerson said, "The mind, once stretched by a new idea, never returns to its original dimensions." One day, Pastor Tony, the worship pastor, asked me to consider co-leading worship on Sunday nights in the new young adults' ministry.

Although I liked having a new challenge to tackle, the idea made me a little nervous. The young adults' group had brought an influx of twenty- and thirty-somethings into the congregation while I was gone. I didn't know many of them, and the prospect of trying to make new friends yet again was daunting.

That first Sunday night before group began, I was running through the set list with Ze, my co-leader, when a guy came in through the back door. He caught my attention because I'd never seen him before, which was unusual at a small-town church. He had blond hair that was starting to thin, and he was wearing Skechers tennis shoes, a dark blue polo shirt, and jeans that were a little bit too big, like no one had ever told him what size fit him best. He made easy conversation with two people near the sound booth. As I watched them talking, I felt a familiar sense of obligation, the *I should go say hi and make the new person comfortable* feeling.

We wrapped up rehearsal. I placed my microphone in the mic stand and made my way down the aisle to say hello, passing the table filled with pizza and vowing to grab a few slices of the three-cheese Alfredo later.

"Hey, you must be new!" I called as I approached him. We both reached out to shake hands. The bracelets around my wrist lightly chimed.

His brow furrowed but his eyes smiled as he replied. "Hi," he said, not offering his name, "I'm most definitely not new here, but you are."

Disarmed and delighted, I laughed. "I guess I am!" I said that I'd been living in Colorado the previous year, so he must've started attending while I was away.

"Ah, that makes sense." He smiled and crossed his arms over his chest. "I heard you singing." He gestured toward the stage. "You're pretty good."

I shrugged and replied casually, "It's a thing I do. I'm Brittany, by the way." I tucked a piece of hair behind my ear and rocked a little on my toes.

"Brady."

"No way!" I clapped my hands, excitement coursing through me. "That was the name of the pastor of the church I attended in Colorado! How crazy is that?"

He gave me that amused little furrowed-brow-and-eye-smile combo again. "Pretty crazy. It's like it's a common name or something," he said dryly. I couldn't tell if he found me amusing or just plain dumb.

I laughed, more at myself than at him, feeling a little silly. "Okay, I'm going to go greet *actual* new people." I inched away.

"How will you know if they're new?"

"As someone recently pointed out, everyone's new to me, so it won't be hard."

He chuckled. "It was nice to meet you, Brittany."

The following Sunday, I saw Brady standing at the back of the auditorium after the group meeting. I made my way out of the sound booth and greeted him with a little smile and wave.

"Nice set tonight," he said.

"Thanks, it's good to see you again." I grabbed a bottle of water off the back table. Brady had on a T-shirt with the Mountain Dew logo, and he was holding a white paper plate with a slice of pizza on it. People milled around us.

"So what do you do, Brady?" I asked.

"I work for a defense contractor," he said.

My eyes lit up. "Oh my gosh, I have always wanted to take karate!" I beamed and took a sip of my water.

He looked at me, confused, then burst into laughter. "No, that's self-defense. I'm an engineer; I work on systems for military vehicles."

"Oh," I responded, half embarrassed, half thinking I'd drawn a completely logical conclusion with the karate comment. "Well, that's way cooler." We were silent for a minute, then both of us burst into laughter. I smiled at him and said, "Do you want to see something crazy?"

"Sure."

I grabbed his hand. "You have to come out to my car. It's nothing weird, I promise."

He followed me into the parking lot, and I opened the back door of my car, where I had stashed some clothes for quick changes between school and work. I pulled out a pair of pants and held them up in the light so he could see the Mountain Dew logos they were covered in.

"It's a sign!" I beamed.

He cocked his head at me, amused. "What's it a sign of?" he asked.

"I don't know." I laughed and pointed at his shirt, which had the Mountain Dew logo on it. "But it means something!"

I should mention that Brady wasn't my usual type; he was actually pretty darn awkward. He had a dry sense of humor, the kind where you never knew if he was being serious or not. He was cute but average-looking, strong but nerdy. He was easy to talk to and fun to be a little flirty with, but there were no sparks, no butterflies; it was just him being him and me being me. We became friends, which was fine with me, since I wasn't actively looking for a relationship.

A couple of weeks later, he made a move. Now, Brady was not a romantic; he was an engineer, a scientist, and he was very practical, even at twenty-three. Instead of inviting me on a date, he organized an outing for the whole group, which was completely out of character for him. But he wanted to "observe" how I interacted with people outside of church, he told me later. If he still liked me after that, he'd take me on a real date.

Of course, I didn't know this then. I just thought he was quirky, which he was. The group dinner went well, and half-way through he leaned over and asked me if he could take me to a movie afterward. I readily agreed, still not quite getting this was meant to be a date.

The movie was unremarkable, but after it, we sat in his truck for nearly *five hours,* talking about everything from our favorite foods to our deepest desires. We told each other about our past relationships and discovered we had both been in ones where we truly believed we were going to marry the other person, and it didn't end up working out. We were similarly serious about looking for a real partnership in a significant other—neither of us was in a rush, but we weren't willing to just play around.

Because of this, we dove into topics most people don't talk about on a first date or even in the first month of a new relationship. We bonded over our shared belief that it was silly to wait to ask where the relationship was going until after you were emotionally invested. Neither one of us was emotionally invested at that point—I wasn't even sure I was attracted to him—but we had an inkling that we might be compatible and we both knew from experience that relationships don't fail because of a lack of love or attraction; they fail because of a lack of compatibility and unmet expectations.

I am a firm believer in telling people how to treat you. I told Brady outright—and with the utmost sincerity—that I believed time was immensely valuable, probably the most valuable thing we possessed, and that I wouldn't take his time for granted and hoped he would respect mine in the same way.

That night we made a pact: As long as we continued to grow in mutual affection, when the time was right, we'd get married. It wasn't romantic; it was logical. And for once, I was glad to just cut through all the nonsense and get real. I wanted to know who Brady was and I wanted to let him see me. If it worked out, great. If not, then it was best not to waste each other's time delaying the inevitable.

That five-hour talk was the best conversation we could have had, because at the end of it, we both recognized an undeniable, nearly perfect level of compatibility. I even wrote in my journal that night, *I don't know—could he be my husband?*

14

Divine Love

Dear Body,

Growing up in the era of rom-coms, I learned there was a formula for love, or at least a good storyline. Girl meets boy; girl likes boy; there's some crazy convoluted plot twist so that girl can't have boy; and then magically a solution appears and they run off into the sunset together. I spent years waiting for a solution that never came because that fantasy was more about loving the idea of someone than about loving the person himself. I had to reconfigure what love was supposed to look like and replace it with what was true: Love is steady, sometimes boring in its normalcy, and often doesn't feel like butterflies but dependability. This type of real, lasting love might not be exciting to watch on Netflix or read about in a book, but it's what we all need.

Body, my story is largely a story about prioritizing need over want and learning to distinguish the *difference between the two. Thank you for supporting me as we continue to navigate this together.*

No relationship is without its challenges. With Chris, love was like a roller-coaster ride of emotion. I was self-conscious, always trying to impress him and worried about saying the wrong thing. Don't get me wrong—there was a time where there was nothing in the world I wanted more than I wanted him, but, like Garth says, "Sometimes I thank God for unanswered prayers."

My relationship with Brady was different. With Brady, love was slow to grow; it felt less like a tidal wave and more like a calm and steady tide gently inching its way higher on the shore as time went on. It was secure, drama-free; it felt mature and patient. There was no hot or cold whirlwind of mixed signals and feelings. There were moments with Brady when I would wonder if the lack of turmoil—the fact that I wasn't bouncing from high highs to low lows—meant that he and I didn't have much passion.

But I was mistaking lack of drama for lack of feeling. Loving him was less of a compulsion and more of a choice. It wasn't a hormone-driven teen romance but a mature relationship built on shared values, admiration, and a willingness to compromise. The more we learned about each other, the more we relaxed in each other's presence, and the more we relaxed, the easier things were.

Over the years, I've thought a lot about these two starkly different types of love. Growing up, I'd believed that if someone doesn't leave your palms sweaty and your heart pounding, it's not true love. But as an adult, I realize that while attraction can fade, it can also develop, and love is largely a choice. My relationship with Brady is the most romantic type of story there is because what could be more romantic than choosing someone over and over again even in the midst of the darkest and most difficult times of your life?

In Greek, there are four different types of love: *eros* (romantic love), *storge* (family love), *philia* (brotherly love), and *agape* (which Christians define as God's divine love). Agape love is the highest form of love. It's the type of love that God has for us; it's unconditional, never changing, always steady. It's the love that originates from God Himself. Whereas these other forms of love may waver, agape love is eternal, and many times it envelops all forms of love in one. That is what I began to build with Brady.

As the months passed, we became even more comfortable with each other. Because I was working three jobs and going to school, we spent most of our time together in the midnight hours. Brady worked the typical nine-to-five, and though we chatted by text throughout the day, when we actually saw each other, it was usually late. At night, we ate pizza, burritos, and fast food, and we rented movies from the local video store, and soon I realized I'd gained a few pounds, because my cute-butt jeans were no longer cute and were 100 percent too tight. They'd slide over my calves without too much tugging, but once I got them up to my thighs, I'd have to dance around, shimmying, shifting, and wriggling from side to side, to get them up, buttoned, and zipped. Shakira was right—hips don't lie, and mine were telling me that I needed new pants.

That weekend, I browsed the racks at JCPenney hoping to find a pair of jeans that I could breathe in. I made my way around the women's clothing section and found nothing that seemed right. I wandered over to the clearance rack and began flipping through the clothes. Suddenly, I spotted something. Not just any something. *The* something.

The most frickin' brilliant thing I had ever seen in my entire life, a pair of jeans with a stretchy panel at the top. I grabbed them from the hanger and ran to the mirror. I could feel my muffin top bulging over the top of my current jeans as I held the stretchy panel jeans up. I couldn't believe what I was seeing. How had I gone my entire life without knowing these glorious pants existed? I tossed them over my forearm and ran back to the rack. There was another brown pair there in a cargo style. I couldn't believe it. I had majorly scored. Pants with Spanx literally built in!

When I got home, I ran into my room, pulled off my old jeans, and slid into the new denim pair. I pulled the panel all the way up—it stopped just below my bra because I'm so short. I pulled my top down over the panel and looked at myself in the mirror. I looked awesome, *and* I was comfortable. I was going to rock those pants every single day.

Later that night, Brady came over to my parents' house and we played around on the trampoline in the backyard. We started to get a little frisky, and when Brady put his hand underneath my shirt, he said, "Wait . . . what do we have here?"

"They're pants!" I yelled. "And they're *amazing*!"

"These are pants? All the way up here?" he said, struggling to find the top.

"Yes! They have this amazing panel that just sucks you right in."

"Brit," he said, laughing, "these aren't *amazing* pants. They're *maternity* pants. For pregnant women."

"Whatever, I don't even care, I got them in every color I could find!"

Brady collapsed on top of me, laughing, and we rolled around on the trampoline beneath the stars like two kids at a sleepover. He pecked me on the nose and said, "If we ever have a daughter, she will only be allowed to wear maternity pants. These things are like Fort Knox—no way I'm getting in there!"

As spring turned to summer, I grew more excited about meeting Brady's family. Brady has a close relationship with his parents and siblings, much like I do with mine, despite our complicated dynamic. The way Brady spoke about his mom and pa had me itching to meet them. I was good with parents, often better than I was with my own peers. Practically speaking, I was set—I was working toward a degree, spending my free time volunteering at church, and living debt-free other than a small car loan that I'd almost paid off. And, hey, Brady adored me. I mean, I was kind of a catch.

At that point, Brady's parents were separated. His mom had moved out after many years of marital turmoil; according to Brady, it had been a long time coming. Brady had helped her move into a renovated barn, not too far from where Brady had grown up, outside of Oklahoma City. His mom invited us, along with his dad, his two sisters—Erica and Aubrey— and his older brother, Michael, to visit for the weekend.

We had a lovely supper together. I kept looking around the table at this big, happy family, feeling really lucky to be there. And the fun continued as the weekend whirled by. His family was charming, and everyone got along so well; we played games, told stories, and spent most of the time laughing. On the drive home I told Brady, "I could see myself calling your parents Mom and Dad."

It wasn't until later, when we were back home and I was hanging at Brady's place, that I realized the weekend might not have gone as well as I'd thought. I overheard a phone conversation between him and his parents, and even though everything he said about me was good, something was off. The emphasis was on all the wrong words.

"She's *great*."

"I *do* love her."

"Yes, I see myself marrying *her*."

When he got off the phone, I inquired softly, my stomach in knots, "Did I do something wrong at your parents' house?"

He hesitated for a moment, then gently said, "No. I think they thought I had a different type, that's all. I guess they envisioned me with somebody different."

"What do you mean?" I asked, crestfallen.

"Well," he continued, "you and I just don't share a lot of the same interests. We are incredibly different people." This was true, but I had a sinking feeling he wasn't telling me everything.

Brady's parents wholeheartedly believed couples should be together for a minimum of two years before they got married. They didn't think we'd known each other long enough to be talking about marriage yet. When Brady asked their opinion of me, they'd shared some concerns.

Those concerns seemed to have less to do with who I was and more to do with how I looked.

Brady's parents told him they saw him with an athletic girl who enjoyed doing outdoorsy things, like camping, hiking, and climbing. At that point, I was pretty heavy—around 215 pounds—and admittedly I wasn't very active, not because I didn't want to be but because it was physically difficult and I was really busy. They cautioned him that people who were obese generally became more so over time, and that led to health issues. They wondered whether he was willing to take all of that on.

I was saddened by Brady's parents' reaction. But my body

was my body. I couldn't transform myself into a waif of a girl in yoga pants and a high ponytail in the blink of an eye. I had been overweight for most of my life, and I didn't see that changing. I also didn't feel like it was something that should be held against me or prevent someone from marrying me. As a parent now, I understand that it's our job to look after and protect our children, and maybe that was all they were trying to do. But as a twenty-year-old woman, all I heard was *They think I'm fat and not good enough for their son.*

They were kind, they were welcoming, but I knew that I wasn't what they wanted for him. I now recognize that their initial response had less to do with me and more to do with their personal issues and the difficulties they'd faced as a couple. But unfortunately, this hindered our relationship for many years. Despite what I'd hoped for, I never started calling them Mom and Dad; they didn't want me to.

Not having their blessing was something I struggled with for about a decade. No matter how hard I tried to impress them, no matter how much weight I lost or how many books I wrote or how many dreams of Brady's I made come true, I still wasn't good enough for him in their eyes.

I had to get to a place within myself where I was so content and proud of who I'd become that I stopped needing their validation. And the most amazing thing happened: When I stopped needing their approval, they finally gave it.

15

Loving What Was

Dear Body,
    I am learning that our ability to heal cannot depend on anyone else's choices. Loving others has fostered the most metamorphic expansion within us, but it hasn't always felt good or easy. In these moments, fear takes hold and begins to whisper to us, "This is going to be like last time" and "They're going to leave you." "You haven't fully recovered from your last heartbreak yet; this one will obliterate you." And sometimes fear can sound like truth.
    So I had to stop listening to the *could bes* and *has beens* and begin to acknowledge what was. I had to override a deep unconscious dread that had been left in the wake of hurt and start to trust in the possibility that not all love stories were the same.

One day, after Brady and I had been together for just five months, he came over to my house, walked into the kitchen, laughed lightly to himself, and said, "So, funny story, I was going to propose to you today."

I turned to face him. "Okay," I said, then paused for a moment before adding, "Then why are we not engaged?" I asked the question in a joking way, but my tummy had started to turn a little. He'd given me a promise ring after we'd been dating for a month and we'd been talking about getting engaged for a while.

"I called my parents to tell them the news, and they felt like we were moving too fast. They think we should slow it down a bit and wait to receive some outside confirmation."

My mind raced. We'd figured we'd get engaged in August, which was already halfway over. We wanted to get married in January, and that would give us six months to plan a wedding; why this change now?

"I thought, why not? It's just a little more time," he said.

His nonchalance triggered my fear response. I'd already spent the past four years of my life caught up with a guy who didn't want the same things out of a relationship as I did. Chris and I had stayed in contact after we broke up. He kept me on the hook by saying things like "I can't find anyone to replace you." He said that his mom could always tell who he was texting because of the way he lit up when he was texting me. She told him she was preparing herself for the day he ran back to Texas to be with me, and she was sure we'd have five babies and be blissfully happy.

After I came back home from Colorado, he suggested that I move to California; we even briefly spoke about getting an apartment together. Chris was the only thing I had ever truly wanted or asked God for. But I knew that if I moved back to California to be with him, I would have to sacrifice the path that I believed God was directing me toward, and I couldn't do it. Because as much as I wanted Chris, I wanted God more.

So for four years, my heart broke continuously as I waited for Chris to come back to me. I had to listen to him talk about the girls he dated and how the relationships never worked out because they weren't me, how we had to take breaks from each other because it was too painful to talk and not be together. And all this time I was completely incapable of moving on because I felt like if I just prayed hard enough and waited long enough, it would all work out in the end.

But it didn't.

When I started talking to Brady, I knew I wouldn't be able to fully commit to a relationship with him while I was still texting and talking to Chris. When I called Chris and told him this, he was sad but he understood. He made one request: If I decided to stop talking to him in order to pursue things with Brady, he wanted that to be it. No more contact—ever. He said that otherwise, he'd just continue to wait by the phone, hoping I'd call, and he needed to know that call was never coming.

I realized that you could have all the love in the world for someone, but love isn't the only ingredient you need for a lasting marriage or a lifelong partnership. So I let him go, and I finally mourned something that had died four years earlier but that neither of us had had the heart to bury. I was terrified I was opening myself up to the same kind of pain with Brady, that he'd keep me on the hook with promises of forever, and although I'd wait patiently, it would all eventually dissolve. It had been so hard to move on from Chris; what if this time I wasn't able to recover?

I'd been confident that Brady and I were on the same page, only to discover his mind was easily swayed by someone else's opinion.

Brady was the first person I'd ever been physical with beyond just kissing. We did things I had never even considered exploring in my previous relationship, things I firmly felt should be reserved for marriage. But we *were* getting married . . . right? Now I wasn't so sure.

Growing up in the 1990s purity culture had really messed with me. My goodness was tied to my virginity, and I believed being sexually immoral—which, in my mind, I had been with Brady—was one of the worst things you could do. But making fear-based choices never produces faith or love. Looking back, I wish that when, or if, I'd made that purity pledge, it was out of love for myself, my future spouse, and the Lord, not because I was afraid He might smite me or that a "good" Christian man or society might not accept me.

It's dangerous when people's acceptance of you hinges on your pleasing them. In that moment, I wasn't sure if I should stay calm and agree to the postponement to please Brady and his parents, urge him to hurry things along so that we could please my parents, or say to hell with all of them and move to New York!

"Brit, it's just a few weeks so they can get used to the idea—"

"So are we going to run every decision we make by your parents first for the rest of our lives? Is your dad going to dictate when we should buy our first house? What about getting pregnant—when is it okay to do that? Will we need his approval then too?" I had officially lost it; I was freaking out. Everything had been fine one moment and gone pear-shaped the next.

I was arrested by fear. I wondered if, by marrying Brady, I was just finding my way into another power-abusing parental-like relationship, one with even more strings and contingencies than I'd dealt with from my own parents. And what about Brady? I'd thought he was his own man. Was he really content to let his parents dictate when he should propose to the girl he claimed to love?

Once I started down this path, I really began spiraling. I'd been perfectly fine before he came along. I'd already sat around waiting for somebody to save me, a knight in shining armor who would rescue me from my parents' house and sweep me off my feet and into a life of marital bliss. But my supposed knight broke me into a million little pieces instead. And here I was, years later, still waiting to be rescued.

I thought I had moved past all that in Colorado. I'd stopped chasing what I thought I wanted so I could walk into what I needed. And yet I was stuck in my parents' house, still trying to navigate the hot-and-cold nature of my relationship with them. Don't get me wrong—I loved them, and I raved about how wonderful they were to anyone who would listen, because they were wonderful. But it was also hard to walk the razor-thin line between the good moments and the bad ones. One moment they were shouting so loudly, I felt like it would bring the roof down, and the next my mom was asking me if I wanted to go with her to get pedicures.

I was on guard all of the time, my fight-or-flight response never turning off but forever hovering at the surface. Coming home after spending a year away from that level of dysfunction was hard. Brady had given me an end date, then casually took it away. If I'd had the finances to move out on my own, I would have, and I feel like that would have alleviated some of my urgency to get married. But I was paying out of my own pocket for my college courses, and the only way I was able to afford it was by not paying rent.

Another major fear of mine was going into debt. My parents had filed for bankruptcy twice while I was growing up; we'd had cars and belongings repossessed and had been evicted from two different homes. I was passionate about not overleveraging myself. If avoiding student loans meant living at home, that was a price I was willing to pay. But without a doubt, it was putting additional pressure on my relationship with Brady.

I felt well and truly stuck. I wanted to marry Brady, but I didn't want to pressure him into something he wasn't ready for. I felt like my back was up against the wall and I wondered where that Colorado girl had gone, the one who didn't need a rescuer, who had discovered that she was capable of saving herself.

Finally, I said, "If you feel like this is what you need to do, I'll give you some time, but you need to know that your time is limited. I'm not just going to sit around waiting indefinitely for you to decide if you want to propose to me or not."

Brady nodded and said, "I understand."

The next four months passed quickly, despite no proposal. Once the initial shock of Brady's "I was going to propose today" confession wore off, my rational mind took over, and I realized that, proposal or not, I wanted this person in my life. My fears were not the only fears on the table and I needed to respect that he had some too. I began to enjoy the space and time between where we were and where I wanted us to be. We decided collectively to pump the brakes a little bit. I put an engagement out of my mind. I opted to focus on school and on carving my own path again; whether that eventually led me to marriage with Brady was still to be seen, but at least I was moving forward.

We both worked long hours and I was going to school full-time, but when we were free, we were inseparable. As an elective that semester, I'd picked up a music-theory class.

That class fed me, giving me a deeper appreciation for the art form that had already given me so much.

Brady knew that if I went to see any symphony outside those required for the class, I would get extra credit. He surprised me with tickets to the Dallas Symphony Orchestra's Christmas concert and told me he was going to take me to a fancy restaurant first. We were both savers, and in lieu of fancy dates, we often chose to stay home and eat frozen burritos or order five-dollar pizzas. So this was out of the ordinary and very special. It would, without a doubt, be the fanciest date I had ever been on. Surprisingly, it was only the third planned date we'd gone on as a couple.

Brady wasn't one for romance or big sweeping gestures of affection. He didn't write me love notes or make me mix tapes; he was just always there. He anchored me in a way that made me feel like I could have both roots and wings. His love was humble, visible in the little things he did, like pulling over to the side of the road to pick me flowers. He took every opportunity to tell me how beautiful he thought I was. He argued with me over politics and philosophy, and he let me be right. And even though it wasn't flashy or showy or Instagram-worthy, his love for me was *loud*.

I bought a new dress for the date; it took hours of searching store after store in the mall to find something my size. I ended up in a bridal store that also carried regular gowns in plus sizes. As I slipped the size 16 black, satiny, formal dress over my head, I could tell that I'd found the one. It was beautiful and made me feel glamorous. And though a hundred dollars was over my budget, I just had to have it. I had blocked off the whole afternoon before the date to get ready. I washed and blow-dried my hair and waved it to perfection. My mom painted my nails purple, and I carefully swiped eyeshadow on my eyelids and blush onto the apples of my cheeks. Finally, I stepped back and looked at myself in the mirror. I felt like a movie star getting ready for a premiere.

As I gathered my things, my phone rang. It was Brady. I looked at the time and assumed he was outside waiting in his car. Instead, he said, "Hey, listen, I'm so sorry. Scott's truck broke down around Adriatica Village. I have to help him and don't want to be late, so can you come and meet me here and we'll head to dinner when I'm done?"

I rolled my eyes. Scott was a good friend of Brady's and he knew this night was special for us. In my eyes, Scott should have called someone else for help. But I pushed the feeling aside and said, "Sure."

"Great," Brady said, "call me when you get here."

I tucked my voluminous skirt around myself in the driver's seat and tried not to wrinkle it as I checked my makeup in the rearview mirror. I had to admit, Adriatica Village was one of my favorite places. It had cobblestoned streets and a path around a huge pond with a fountain in the middle and a chapel, although that wasn't finished yet. I figured if I got there and Brady was still working on Scott's truck, I could just walk around a bit and explore.

When I got there, I dialed Brady's number.

"Hey!" Brady answered. "We're just about done. We're on the other side of the bell tower; just meet us here."

"Okay, I'm coming." I laughed. Something about Brady's voice sounded so light and airy, I could tell he was excited about the date too.

As I walked around the bell tower, I noticed a large book on the steps, leaning against a railing. The book was covered in sunflowers and had a picture in the middle. As I got closer to it, I realized it was a picture of me. I picked up the book and carefully opened it to the first page. Brady had penned a beautiful love letter that began with "Come away with me on this magical journey where two hearts become one." He'd filled the book with drawings of different landscapes and mystical houses in the sky, under the sea, and even one on a faraway planet—all drawn by hand. He invited me to come along with him on the journey of a lifetime where we could build a home in each other. On the last page of the book it said, "This is where I am going, will you go with me? If yes, shout and wave toward the chapel."

So I did.

Nothing happened.

I jumped up and down and shouted again. "Hey! Brady!" I called, feeling silly.

Still nothing happened.

Finally, I flipped over the last page of the book. On the other side it said, "Don't see me? Turn around."

I turned around and there was Brady, kneeling, with an obscenely massive ring box. He opened it to reveal a *giant* fake ring that he had whittled out of a block of wood! I doubled over with laughter. He smirked, satisfied that his joke had paid off.

He placed it on my finger, laughing. I couldn't even hold my hand up, it was so heavy. I was laughing so hard my entire body was shaking.

"No, no, I'm just kidding," he said as he slid the massive ring off my finger and gave me my real ring. The real ring, which Brady had spent months saving up for, had a beautiful, one-half-carat round-cut diamond set in an exquisitely dainty Neil Lane band.

My parents, who had been hiding in the bell tower filming the whole time, came down and excitedly hugged and kissed us. They gushed over the ring and the proposal and said they felt lucky to be the first to congratulate us.

We made our way to the restaurant for an extravagant

dinner, then went to the symphony. I looked around the lobby of the concert hall and giggled. With me in my ball gown and Brady in his suit, we were far more dressed up than anyone else there, but I didn't care. I was having the night of my life. When we sat, Brady reached over, grabbed my hand, and whispered, "I love you." As the lights dimmed and the music swelled, I realized that Brady was right—all the waiting hadn't really mattered.

Loving after you've been hurt can feel like an exercise in learning how to trust again. I wanted so desperately to control the timeline of our love and how Brady responded in certain situations, but I now know I was trying to control the situation because I was afraid. Trusting someone is the ultimate way of saying "I love you."

Love will never be anew like that first time, naïveté trying to convince you that you are impervious to heartbreak as you jump off into the unknown. Loving again is loving from experience, and that can be scary and hard and eye-opening.

When I fell in love with Brady, I made sure to fall in love with the Brady that existed in that moment—not the person I envisioned him being in the future, but the person who was right in front of me. I had spent so much time loving versions of people that never existed that I'd missed loving the ones who were staring me in the face, and I swore that I would stop romanticizing all that could be and begin to love what was.

16

We Do

Dear Body,
    When I was younger, the world seemed black-and-white to me. There were things I believed and choices I made based entirely on other people's convictions in a desperate grab for morality. It was easier to be led to their truth than to seek it on my own. So when I committed "the ultimate sin," I was surprised that I didn't feel ashamed about it at all. It's easier to see the world in two colors than in the vibrant Technicolor that it is. This is how I began to dismiss the belief that you, my body, were dangerous. A new seed was planted: the idea that I could actually learn to love you.

Although we weren't yet married by Christmas of that year, Brady and I split holiday time between our families and got a taste of what married life might be like. We celebrated Christmas Eve with my parents and then drove three hours to be with Brady's parents.

It was my first Christmas away from my family, so seeing the traditions and dynamics of another family was new and exciting. I am not someone who holds grudges or goes into a tailspin over conflict. I know that in the long run, it will do more harm to me to spend time in anger or hurt. I welcomed this holiday as a fresh start of sorts—I was going to let go of my feelings about Brady's parents' first impression of me and hold on to the wonderful things about their family: how playful and generous they were, the fact that they didn't have much but what they had, they were happy to share, how his dad could have a conversation with anyone and his optimism was contagious, and the way his mom was the ultimate hostess and wellness advocate.

Christmas with Brady's family was different from my family's Christmas. For one, Brady and all of his siblings were adults, so for the first time in my life I was able to experience an adults-only Christmas. We exchanged gifts, ate a delicious meal, and instead of the TV blaring or kids shouting, we spent a relatively quiet evening playing board games and having inspiring conversations. It couldn't have gone better.

Brady's older brother was getting married on January 1, and we were both invited to be part of the wedding, so we stayed in Brady's childhood bedroom after Christmas. On New Year's Eve, we all had a little bit of champagne to ring in 2011. After the ball dropped, his parents went to bed. Brady and I quietly retreated to his old bedroom. The champagne had us giggling, and our hands began to wander. Up to that point, Brady and I had been physical with each other, but we'd always maintained boundaries. There was something different about that night. It wasn't the champagne, because I'd barely had two sips, but I felt drunk off his kisses and the magic of the coming new year. It felt right; I didn't want to wait anymore, so we stopped waiting.

As wrong as I'd always been told that it was, it didn't feel wrong at all. I suspect it's because when I said yes to his proposal, I had already declared my intention. We didn't intend to have a trial period where we tried married life on for size. As far as I was concerned, a trial period was just a way of making a perpetual habit out of never fully committing to anyone. I didn't need a wedding ceremony, a big white dress, or a document from the state to tell me what I already knew. The second I said yes to his proposal, I was saying yes to all of it.

On the drive back to my parents' house, I texted them and told them I was staying an extra night at Brady's parents' in Oklahoma City. Really, though, we drove straight through and I stayed with him overnight at his apartment. I was twenty-one and it was the first time I'd ever lied to them about a boy.

Brady felt worse about it than I did. "We've got to get married soon. I don't like lying to your parents, and this isn't what the Lord would want."

I shrugged. "We've already been through premarital counseling, we already have our marriage license, I know plenty of pastors . . . heck, we could get married this weekend."

He immediately seized on the idea. "Yeah, we could! Truthfully, it'll be hard to hold the line now that we've crossed it. I just want to make sure we do this right. I don't want to taint our relationship with lies and sneaking around."

"You're a real gentleman, Brady Williams, wanting to make an honest woman out of the likes of me," I joked. "I think you're very sweet. Plus, think of all the money we'll save and stress we'll avoid!"

Saturday, January 8, was the original wedding date we'd chosen before we postponed getting engaged. Now we decided, why not just go for it? That would give us six days to put together a fun, easy, nontraditional wedding.

My parents were excited to jump right into the planning.

If we were going to get married in their living room, it was going to be the most beautiful living-room wedding anyone had ever seen! Everybody else hopped on board too. Aunt Kim and my mom practically bought out Hobby Lobby—no artificial sunflower or votive candle was safe. My grandma made our wedding cake—three tiers of absolute perfection—and altered an off-the-rack wedding dress I'd found less than forty-eight hours before the wedding.

Wedding-dress shopping had not gone at all the way I'd envisioned—me surrounded by girlfriends, drinking champagne, all of us laughing and crying as I tried on one gorgeous ball gown after another. Instead, it was just my mom and me running all over town trying to find an off-the-rack dress that fit me and was within our price range.

The first place we went didn't carry anything in a size 16, which is funny, considering it's one of the most common dress sizes in America. I tried on one dress that was outrageously priced and that I had no hope of ever buttoning up. I felt humiliated and embarrassed; it was clear that I wasn't going to be able to fit into a single one of these dresses and I prayed that other shops would have larger sizes.

We abandoned the fancy boutique and tried David's Bridal; they had one dress in a size 12. Even though it was two sizes too small, I tried it on, and again I felt like an ogre. There wasn't even a prayer that the back would zip up. My mom called my grandma to see if she could meet us, because maybe she could alter it? I checked the price tag—it was four hundred dollars, twice as much as we'd budgeted for the dress.

"Mom," I said quietly as she was talking to my grandma on the phone, explaining all the alterations the dress would need. "It's too expensive, it needs too much work, it's not meant to be."

Holding her hand over the receiver, she asked, "Are you sure?"

"Yes," I said, "it's not the one."

My mom had the clerk put the dress on hold anyway, "just in case."

There was one more shop on our list, a place where a girlfriend of mine had found her off-the-rack dress for way under retail. I wasn't hopeful that anything would fit. I had already resolved to wear either my black engagement dress or a white sundress I'd picked up at Forever 21, but my mom was adamant that I get married in a nice white wedding dress.

I became cautiously optimistic when we entered the third shop. My mom explained our situation to the lady at the counter and discreetly asked if she had anything in my size. I didn't want to waste an hour browsing racks of dresses I'd never have a prayer of fitting into. The saleslady said, "I think I have just the thing!"

Moments later, she brought out a strapless, tiered mermaid gown in off-white. "This is a size fourteen but it has a lace-up back, so there's wiggle room!" It was $299 but my mom waved my worry away and said the price didn't matter.

I tried it on, and it fit like a glove. It wasn't my dream dress, but at that point I was just happy to find something that fit. Even all these years later, it still makes me sad that this was my experience and that it remains the experience of many plus-size people around the world. Stuck wearing whatever fits instead of choosing what you love most.

The saleslady kindly offered to give us a discount on the dress so that it was closer to our price range, and it felt like a sign that I was on the right path. We drove straight to my grandma's and she met us with her pincushion in hand; she folded up the bottom of the dress and laughed about how she'd have to cut six inches off to get it the right length. But my grandma is a miracle worker, and she bent over backward to get the dress finished and the wedding cake done on time.

Even Brady's family was supportive. I was surprised his parents didn't try to stop the quick wedding, but Brady said, "You have to understand, the engagement was the thing for them. I've already promised that I'm going to marry you, I've already declared my intentions. It doesn't matter when the wedding is."

And it was a good thing it didn't matter, because, as planned, six days later, we had a small, humble wedding in my parents' living room. It was officiated by the worship pastor who'd been my mentor for all those years. It was an intimate affair—immediate family only—and it was utterly perfect.

17

Settling In

Dear Body,

Over the years, I've discovered that timing is everything and plans are easily disrupted. I used to follow a road map that I thought was the key to living a fulfilled and successful life, but just about every plan I made for myself was upset somewhere along the way. I thought I knew what was best for me and my life because I'd observed what seemed best for others. I think Proverbs 16:9 says it beautifully: "We can make our plans, but the Lord determines our steps." I am grateful to be living a life composed of surprise and unplanned blessings, one where I make plans but often end up changing direction, always ending up right where I'm supposed to be.

As Brady and I settled into marriage, we decided that we were going to wait to have kids. I wanted to finish up school, and because we'd gotten married so fast, we thought it would be nice to have a few years for just the two of us. Brady wanted to save up for a down payment on a house and create a homestead (he has a farmer's soul) before we added children to the mix. I wanted to travel, see the world, and experience all of the things that life had to offer. We were only twenty-one and twenty-four; we had our whole lives to start a family.

Our sex life was good, but there were desires that both of us kept hidden in the beginning. This wasn't intentional, but I think, like any relationship, there is a refining and maturing that must take place, a trust that has to develop during intimacy. While we were satisfied with each other at the time, I don't know that either of us realized there was room to grow, and I'm glad that we didn't. It's made exploring and expanding our sexual relationship over the years that much more exciting.

Birth control was a challenge. I absolutely did not want to take hormonal contraception; I worried about the possible side effects. Initially, we tried spermicide, but it kept giving me UTIs, and Brady hated how condoms interfered with sensitivity. I researched tirelessly—it's my nature—and I finally came to the conclusion that there wasn't a single form of manufactured birth control that I was comfortable with. (Years later, I would discover the fertility awareness method and natural family planning, which is what I continue to use today to avoid pregnancy.)

Brady finally offered a thought. "In the Bible, there were women who didn't get pregnant for years and years because the Lord just didn't want them to be pregnant. It wasn't because they weren't sexually active; it just wasn't time yet. So maybe we just pray to the Lord and let Him know that we would like not to be pregnant for two years, and then if it happens, it happens. If we get pregnant, we'll just take that as a sign from the Lord that we were supposed to have kids sooner than we thought."

It was better than anything I'd come up with. So that evening, we prayed about it, putting our contraception in the Lord's hands.

I got pregnant that weekend. Although it was a shock and kind of hilarious to find out I'd gotten pregnant so quickly, and while it wasn't what I'd envisioned for myself at this stage of my life, in my family, it was all I had known. Having children that young wasn't my plan, but it was familiar.

I'm deeply romantic at heart, and I had spent years fantasizing what life would look like at this point. For the first couple of months, I leaned into this vision of marital bliss. I cooked five-star dinners, packed sexy little notes in his lunches, and got up early to make him breakfast in bed on the weekends. I made keeping up with work and school look easy as I planned fun things and activities for us to do. I had a Pinterest board dedicated to "couple goals" and I was determined to be a wife he could never complain about.

When I was growing up, my parents—who sometimes viewed me more as a friend than a child—would complain about each other to me. At the time, this made me feel grown up and important, but it actually sowed a deep-seated fear that one day my spouse would speak poorly of me behind my back as well. My mother tended to dominate the relationship, and my dad resented that; I didn't want Brady to ever resent me. As a result, I tried to make myself smaller, perfect, pin-worthy so Brady would never be displeased with me.

But all of this changed when I was about six weeks pregnant and I started having awful, debilitating nausea that lasted all day. I was barely able to do anything. I couldn't be in the car, I couldn't look at a computer screen, I couldn't *move* without vomiting. For a while, I tried to continue on like nothing had changed. I had to be up at four thirty A.M. to make it to my six A.M. class, pulling over several times on the drive to throw up. On rare occasions, I made it to the lecture hall on time, but even then, I had to leave three to four times during the lecture to throw up. Finally, I admitted to myself that what I was doing wasn't working and I withdrew from my classes.

Thankfully, at that point, I had a nannying job that was sedentary. I was working with a little boy I loved, Levi, who was born with MECP2 duplication syndrome. (MECP2 is a rare genetic condition that affects mostly males and results in moderate to severe intellectual disability, weak muscle tone, feeding difficulties, and speech delays.) I was able to keep my job working with him, remaining still while taking him through speech-therapy lessons and dexterity exercises. It was a job that allowed me to be sick when I was and strong when I could be. Levi's mom was amazing—supportive, nurturing, and fine with letting me journey through my pregnancy while working with her precious boy. She even offered to let me bring the baby with me after I gave birth, which was beyond generous.

Although I was able to hold on to my job, I started to slip and let all the house stuff—the cooking and cleaning and homemaking—that had once seemed vital fall through the cracks. My food aversions were so strong that I couldn't cook. My energy levels were so low that I wasn't keeping up with the laundry or any of the cleaning. I even began to neglect my personal hygiene. When I was home, I was really just living between the bathroom and the couch all day.

I could feel Brady's frustrations rise as our apartment became messier and more chaotic. I could tell that he didn't understand that I wasn't just really lazy, that I was indeed very sick, and not at all myself during pregnancy. Because of our premarital counseling sessions, I knew that unmet expectations are a major factor in most relationship issues, so I decided to ask Brady how he was feeling. One night when he got home from work, I sat him down and asked him about it directly. "Are you angry with me?"

"I'm not angry," he said, "I'm just frustrated. I know you're sick but when things aren't tidy, my irritation level rises. It's not even a conscious thing; clutter just gets under my skin, and the apartment . . . well, it's been—"

"Oh, it's a pigsty, I know," I said. I'd been letting the dishes pile up for days; new-baby stuff had overtaken the dining room; my clothes were strewn everywhere. I explained to him that this situation wasn't permanent, but for the moment, I couldn't continue to hit the bar I'd set for myself. Up to that point, Brady had not truly realized how sick I was. "I can't manage it all right now. I know I said I've got it, but I don't got it. I need help."

And just like that, Brady's frustration melted away. He had an expectation that I wasn't capable of fulfilling at that point, and he was receptive and understanding when I explained that things had changed. He was more than happy to help when he realized that I wasn't just being negligent but that I was physically incapable of doing all that I'd been doing before. I wasn't imagining exhaustion, I wasn't feigning sickness, and I wasn't using pregnancy as an excuse; my body needed something and I was listening. Being open with Brady about those needs, communicating about how they affected him, and sharing honest dialogue offered so much relief.

Cleaning the kitchen and preparing the meals became Brady's job, since the worst of my triggers were in the kitchen.

He urged me to take it easy and rest, so I let most of the household stuff go, only really keeping up with the laundry. This was our first trial as a married couple, and I felt really proud of the way we communicated through it instead of letting the frustration fester. I hoped that it was an indicator of things to come.

18

Best-Laid Plans

Dear Body,
I have often felt betrayed by you. In sickness,
in pregnancy, in birth, and in life. Women's bodies
are designed to bring life into the world, and I was
surrounded by women who were successful at it. You
let me down.

Birthing babies was in my blood. My mom had seven healthy pregnancies with no issues except for a breach presentation with her seventh baby, my brother Tristan, her only C-section. My grandma had six healthy vaginal deliveries. I had aunts, friends, and mentors who were all masters at the art of pregnancy and birth. They made it look innate, effortless, and I never doubted for a moment that I would be a natural at it too.

So when I saw those double pink lines, there was never any fear or turmoil, just pure ecstatic joy and excitement. A deep calmness emanated from within me; I felt that I was born to do this and do it well.

A character trait of mine is that when I get turned on to a subject, I research it to the point of exhaustion. It becomes all I talk about and think about, and I want everyone else to know about it too. I began to devour documentaries like *The Business of Being Born* and immersed myself in books like Ina May Gaskin's *Ina May's Guide to Childbirth* and *Spiritual Midwifery*. I wrote a birth plan and took classes. All of my research led me to one important decision: I would have an unmedicated, natural hospital birth.

In my mind, I was a healthy twenty-one-year-old woman. I did not view my morbid obesity and the fact that I ultimately gained seventy additional pounds during my pregnancy as issues that placed me in a high-risk category. My mom also birthed babies while overweight, and a dear friend of mine was over three hundred pounds and had had several successful home births.

There have been times in my life where I neglect the forest for the trees; this was one of those times. I was so focused on learning everything I could and preparing for labor and birth that I neglected my body. When the horrible all-day nausea began at six weeks, my focus wasn't on improving my nutrition but on simply keeping food down.

I lived on a steady diet of ginger ale, Preggie Pops, Flamin' Hot Cheetos, chicken tenders, and peanut butter sandwiches. It wasn't until years later that I discovered my all-day pregnancy nausea was a signal my body was sending me that it wasn't getting the things that it needed—namely protein, natural folate, and fiber. Nutritional requirements, of course, vary widely and differ greatly for everyone. For me, it turns out, these nutrients were essential.

I went into labor at thirty-nine weeks. Early labor was simple—the contractions were soft, a tightening around my belly that released gently after a few moments. My grandma, who was a labor and delivery nurse, lived right down the street, so she came over and checked me in the early hours of the morning. I was one and a half centimeters dilated. She told me I had a long way to go, so I should start walking to get things moving, but it was the end of November in Texas, the day before Thanksgiving, and freezing cold outside. We told Brady to go off to work, and my mom took me to the mall so we could walk the baby out in a heated place.

About forty-five minutes into our walk, my stomach began to growl, and my mom promised me that after another lap around, we'd grab a Cinnabon to share. Halfway through our last lap, we stopped at the bathroom and I discovered bright red blood in my underwear. My mom strongly suggested that we head to the hospital "just to get checked." A NICU nurse, well versed in all of the things that potentially could go wrong, my mom was always going to err on the side of caution.

I called Brady on the drive to the hospital and told him that I would probably get sent home because I was still in very early labor, but he decided to take off work and come anyway. We said "I love you" and five minutes later, my mom parked in front of the hospital. She spoke with the receptionist at the front desk and showed her badge; I was ushered back into L and D within minutes. They got me in a gown and strapped a fetal heart monitor around my belly. My mom and the L and D nurse watched the monitor. The nurse asked me to roll onto my left side. After a moment, she requested that I turn onto my right as she placed an oxygen mask on my face. She slipped out of the room, and I asked my mom if she thought everything was okay. She smiled and tried to reassure me, but I got the sense that something was very wrong.

A moment later, the nurse entered the room with two more nurses in tow. One of them approached me and said they were admitting me and that I needed to sign a few forms. Another came around to the other side of the bed and told me she was going to begin an IV. I saw my mom pick up her phone and whisper, "Where are you? Get here now." The first nurse put on protective surgery garb as she said, "We just paged your doctor, she is going to be here any moment." She motioned to the monitor. "See this line here? That is your contraction. And see that line there? That is the baby's heartbeat. You can see with every contraction the heart rate goes down and after the contraction is over, it never comes back up and recovers. We're going to have to perform a cesarean."

Dumbfounded and suspicious, I looked to my mom for confirmation, wondering if all this could be true. I felt fine, I was healthy, I had a plan. "Are you sure?" I asked her softly, tears in my eyes. "I don't want to have surgery, that wasn't my plan."

A moment later, Brady came rushing into the room. I had monitors hooked up everywhere, oxygen, IVs—his deeply concerned and piercing blue eyes met mine as a nurse handed him a bright yellow surgical garment and told him to suit up quickly. My doctor came in, already dressed for surgery. I didn't know what to think; I knew that there were probably questions I should ask but I couldn't formulate the words to ask any of them. My eyes kept leaking, I couldn't stop my body from shaking, and the room was a blur of activity as everyone prepared for surgery.

Brady gripped my hand and kissed my head. "It's going to be okay," he said.

But in my heart, I didn't feel like it was going to be. I'd

read all the books, I'd done all the research, I'd come up with a plan—how could something go wrong? How could I fail?

"I know it's not ideal," my doctor said, her eyes narrowing with concern, "but this is what has to happen. We're going to take you back to surgery and get this baby out."

While no one dared say it as they wheeled me through the halls of the unit into the ice-cold, stark white operating room, this was an emergent situation; we'd been watching my baby nearly die on that monitor.

When we got to the OR, I had a difficult time keeping my body still so they could position the epidural. This godsend of a nurse held me as my body shook. I wish I could remember her name; I can't, but I can distinctly remember the way that she smelled, like warmth and home and peace.

"I'm scared," I said. I quietly cried into her shoulder.

"It isn't fair," she whispered into my hair as she bore the weight of my body while the anesthesiologist readied my back. "But this is what mamas do. We adapt and we do our best to care for the tiny ones we've been entrusted with. You are so strong; you don't even know how strong you are yet. But you're about to find out. I can tell that you're an amazing mother already. Your baby's not even here yet and you care so much about its safety and well-being. The baby is so lucky to have you, and even though this wasn't your plan, there will be good that comes out of it, I promise." She kissed my hair and calmed me down like a sister or a friend or, really, a mother.

I lay back on the table with Brady by my side, and moments later, our daughter was born.

"Oh, she's tiny!" my doctor exclaimed.

"She's beautiful," one of the nurses commented and all the other nurses muttered in agreement.

"What a doll! We're just going to take her over to the warmer, Mama."

They held her up so that I could see her: Availeth, our baby girl, named for the scripture James 5:16: "The fervent effectual prayer of a righteous man availeth much." She *was* tiny. But she was okay, and I tried to convince myself that that was all that really mattered. Even though it was the standard response when people heard about our emergency birth situation—"She's okay, that's all that matters"—at the time, it frustrated me, because I felt in my weary spirit that it *wasn't* the only thing that mattered, and saying that it was somehow trivialized my grief instead of acknowledging and validating it.

They kept Avey and me separate for a time and I had a reaction to the anesthesia. I couldn't stop my body from shaking or my teeth from chattering, and I was freezing. Fifteen minutes after I'd been wheeled to recovery, a nurse came around the corner cradling Avey, all wrapped up in a hospital blanket with a pink cap. She was holding Avey in one arm, and in her other hand she held a bottle. She was feeding her.

I sat up a little straighter and said through chattering teeth, "Oh, I'm sorry, I was going to breastfeed her. We weren't planning to use formula." The nurse shook her head. "Her blood sugar is really low, Mama, and we need to get it up. If we can't get it up through a feed, we're going to have to put her on an IV and a feeding tube. I promise, this is the best option right now, since you aren't producing milk yet."

I felt very disoriented and confused, like I was existing in an alternate reality or a dream state. I felt very, very young, too young to have a sick baby, too young to have given birth, too young to understand let alone navigate what I was feeling. I had a million questions. I managed to ask if she was okay and was told again that her blood sugar and temperature were low.

"Can I hold her?" I asked.

"Of course, if you're feeling up to it!" The nurse handed her to me, cautioning that she was going to have to take her temperature in a few minutes, and if Avey couldn't start regulating her own temperature, they'd have to take her to the NICU to get warm. Although she was a full-term baby, she was only five pounds, one ounce. She felt so delicate in my hands. I asked if they could put her on me, skin to skin, so that I could try to warm her up, and they did. They laid her on my chest under all the blankets and sheets.

I felt a little awkward cradling her against my bare chest for the first time. I was still cold myself and kept asking them to layer heated blankets on top of us. I was too nervous to try to nurse her and felt like I needed to ask permission to even breathe around her. She didn't feel like mine; she felt like she belonged to them, and I was just in the way. When they took her temperature again, they told me they had to take her to the NICU because she just wasn't warm enough. I got to hold her for about five minutes before they took her across the hall.

About an hour later, nurses took me back to my room, but first they wheeled me into the NICU in my hospital bed, Brady walking next to me. Avey was in the incubator, all curled up, with little sensors on her so they could monitor her. She was getting oxygen from a nasal cannula and was under a heat light. They said we couldn't touch her but we could take a picture with her, so we did. We were in there for only a couple minutes before my nurse told me that it was time to get me settled in my own room. I asked when I could see her again and the nurse told me that I wouldn't be able to come back until visiting hours tomorrow when I was up and walking. Maybe after breakfast.

I looked at the clock. It was only four P.M.

Tomorrow was Thanksgiving.

How sad that she would have to spend her first Thanksgiving morning all alone.

When Brady and I were finally in my room, I couldn't stop the tears.

"It's the strangest thing," I said as the tears made dark little spots on my white hospital sheet, "I feel like we never had a baby at all. Like my entire pregnancy, all of it, was just a dream, and here I am waking up from a ten-month slumber, grieving a baby I never really had. Was it all a dream? Am I dreaming?"

At some point that evening, my doctor came to visit and talk us through what had happened earlier.

"If you had arrived an hour later, it would have been a different outcome. We saved a baby today. I had your placenta sent to pathology. In thirty years of obstetric gynecology, I have never seen a placenta like that. We won't know until we get the report back, but I'm pretty sure it ruptured and that was part of the issue."

I wondered if the rupture was the source of the bright red blood I'd seen in the bathroom. I was so grateful for my mom's insistence that I get to the hospital. It seemed the outcome would have been devastating if we hadn't.

"Will we be able to have more kids?" Brady asked.

"I highly recommend that Brittany focus on getting healthy and losing weight before attempting any more pregnancies. Morbidly obese mothers have a much higher risk of complications. She needs to lose a hundred pounds, minimum, before I'd see her as a patient again."

I'd gained nearly seventy pounds while I was pregnant

with Avey; I was around two hundred and eighty pounds when I gave birth. I knew I wasn't the picture of health, but I'd never imagined that my weight could affect my pregnancy. I wondered if this body had caused this outcome or if it was just a fluke. My doctor had left me with little comfort and made me feel ashamed, like I was clearly the one to blame.

The NICU made my bonding with Avey strange and tricky. It was odd to ask somebody's permission to do things with your own baby. It created a continuation of the feeling that it was all a dream; she wasn't mine. My first motherly experience was watching nurses change her diaper as I worked up the courage to ask, "Can I help? Is that allowed?" I felt timid, like I was a nuisance, someone who was just making their jobs harder.

The on-call pediatrician explained to us that Avey had extremely low platelet levels and they couldn't figure out why they were so low. Her blood sugar was also incredibly low, which was part of the reason she couldn't regulate her body temperature. For a while, going to the NICU left us with more questions than answers. Every time we visited, she had something new hooked up to her. On our first visit, she had a nasal cannula; next came a feeding tube, an IV, and a humidity hood. Eventually she required blood platelet transfusions.

Was it genetic? The endocrinologist thought she might have a very rare blood clotting disorder. All three of us underwent various tests to rule out anything and everything.

During this time, I had to check out of the hospital and Avey had to stay. Leaving without her, making the drive every day to sit by her bedside and deliver breast milk—none of it looked like I'd thought having a baby would. My heart was heavy, but I didn't feel like I was allowed to be sad, because she was alive, right? And not everyone was as lucky as we were. I was sleep-deprived, exhausted, and still recovering from surgery. Pumping every two hours became a religion, and it was clear I was struggling with a bit of postpartum depression. I was also harboring a secret I kept from everyone, something I was so deeply disturbed by and ashamed of that I couldn't even find a voice for it.

I didn't feel like she was mine.

I would hold her and she was beautiful, but I felt like I was holding someone else's baby. I waited for it to feel like the books said it would—this instantaneous connection and bond—but it wouldn't come.

After a couple of weeks in the hospital, she made a miraculous recovery, and all of her issues were chalked up to malnourishment at birth. When she came home, I spent days in bed with her, skin to skin, never leaving her for a moment, because I wanted to feel something, anything. I kept reaching out and finding nothing but sadness. And then I would feel terrible for feeling sadness, and then I would hate myself because what kind of person did that make me? Something was wrong with me. She was literally perfect, but she felt like a stranger.

She wouldn't breastfeed, so I had to pump. Pumping made things so much worse. Huddled in our dark apartment, day in and day out, I couldn't leave because of my rigid pumping schedule. I continued to pump every two hours because no one told me that when your milk comes in, you can begin to scale back a little. I even set alarms in the middle of the night. We were drowning in breast milk, and I felt like my entire life had been reduced to my capacity as a milk cow.

When would I feel like a mom?

When Avey was a month old, I finally broke. I told Brady, "I can't do this anymore. I have to stop pumping entirely or I have to get her to take the breast. I can't do this thing where I'm pumping, cleaning, and then feeding. It's driving me crazy."

Brady took three days off work and stayed home with me to help get her to nurse. The lactation consultants at the hospital told me that at one month, having been on a bottle for her entire life, Avey was just not going to breastfeed. But I firmly believed she would not let herself starve. So Brady and I did what every rational couple does in a time of crisis: We turned to YouTube. We watched about a billion different videos and became convinced we could do it by using Avey's natural instincts.

We were determined, yet every time I tried, she would not latch on correctly. It was the most painful, excruciating process, and every step we took seemed to make the pain worse while Avey made little to no progress. This went on for three days. In between breastfeeding attempts, we'd been feeding her with a syringe so that she was never starving. We finally found the one video we needed: It reminded the mother to gently break a baby's suction before removing her from the breast. It turns out that was the missing piece. If she latched incorrectly, I would gently stick my finger between her mouth and my breast to break suction, before repositioning her to try to latch again. My nipples were cracked, bleeding, and raw but learning how to break suction enabled us to work on improving her latch without tremendous pain. It took three days of adjustment, trial and error, tears and frustration, but she eventually took to it and started nursing like a pro. We were elated and I was exhausted. But we were both so glad to be over this first hurdle.

I was told by lactation consultants that it was completely unheard-of for a baby to start nursing after a month of bottle-feeding. They'd told us we'd never be able to make it happen. Later, I would learn that I'd been misinformed by these consultants, that it was not impossible, just more difficult. It was nonetheless still a tremendous accomplishment. Brady was there taking care of me, making sure I ate, tending to the house, and acting as a stand-in lactation consultant. Without his coaching and support, I don't know that we would have been able to do it. This was a turning point for all three of us. Breastfeeding created the bond I felt had been missing, and we were all much more content. Pumping was one of the most difficult things I had ever done, and I gained so much respect for mothers who pump for their babies. It is truly a selfless act of love. I also gained new understanding for those who choose not to breastfeed or pump at all. Experiencing such a dramatic life change, adding a whole new person to the family, and on top of that assuming a new identity as a food source is mentally, physically, and emotionally draining for the mother. There should never be any stigma or shame surrounding how parents choose to feed their little ones.

Even though things got easier at that point, I still struggled with the loss of what I'd envisioned the birth of my first baby and my entry into motherhood would look like. Even if it could have been worse, I still had to grieve the loss of my plan.

Brady said, "I can't even begin to imagine how you feel, but I do know that it wasn't fair and that it hurt you very deeply, and for that I am so sorry."

Validation. Acceptance.

For so long, I felt like speaking the words aloud would be a trespass against Avey. To say that I'd had a hard time bonding, even though she was beautiful and perfect, made me feel like even more of a failure as a mother. But the bond came. The healing was slow, but it came too. And talking about it didn't hurt; it helped.

Through all this, I learned so much about myself. I learned

that in moments of crisis, strangers can be like angels. I learned that grief isn't just about mourning a death; it's about processing the pain of loss in any form, and processing was vital for me. Most important, I realized that I could do hard, seemingly impossible things.

Little did I know how important that realization would come to be.

19

Eating, Naturally

Dear Body,
* I wasn't always fair to you in what I gave you for*
sustenance—mentally, emotionally, or physically.
As a result, you weren't always fair to me. As we've
gotten older, we've come to a deeper understanding
of each other. I am beginning to take accountability
for the role that I've played.

Brady's mom was really into aromatherapy, nutrition, gut health, and whole-body wellness. She was a wealth of information on healing, detoxing, and all the components that go into a balanced lifestyle. Brady has therefore always been a holistic, natural guy. He loves to be outside, prefers organic, non-GMO foods, and is careful about the things he puts in (and even on) his body.

Brady was the only man I'd ever met who actually ate *real* food regularly. When I went over to his house for the first time, he had fruits and vegetables in his refrigerator. I didn't even know what to do with that; I blurted out, "You're so healthy," then added with a flirty wink, "Who *are* you?"

As wild as it seems to me now, I'd never really put together that some foods were better for you than others. I was raised on a processed, nutrient-starved diet. I mistakenly believed I was incredibly healthy if I ate a banana once a week, because—fruit. When Brady and I began dating, it wasn't obvious to me that we had such different lifestyles because we were always grabbing and going or both exhausted after a day of work. Our meals were about indulgence and convenience; little thought was given to food beyond that.

The very first time we ever went shopping as a married couple, I nonchalantly grabbed a ninety-seven-cent loaf of white bread off the shelf, the cheapest option, and threw it in the cart. Brady looked at me in shock, completely horrified, as if I'd just committed a crime. I don't think the guy had eaten a slice of white bread in his life—his mom had always purchased whole wheat or they'd made it themselves.

Brady looked at the bread in the cart, then back at me, confused, and asked, "What are you doing?"

"Buying bread," I responded, confused myself. "It's on the list!"

"I wouldn't call that bread." He chuckled lightly while grabbing the bread from the cart. "Can I show you something?"

I nodded, not realizing I was about to get my first lesson in label reading.

He pulled a loaf of what my siblings and I referred to as "yucky brown bread" off the shelf and showed me the ingredients side by side with the white bread's—unbleached flour versus bleached enriched flour, the grams of sugar in each, the names of these sugars, and the added vitamins in one versus the naturally occurring vitamins in the other. He explained that manufacturers added synthetic vitamins and fortified or enriched the bread to bulk it up because they stripped every-thing out of it when they bleached the flour. It's essentially dead food, completely devoid of nutrition. It does nothing for the body; it's simply empty calories. I appreciated that Brady was gentle about telling me this. He didn't need me to agree with him; he was just offering information.

"This is the one we want because these ingredients are better for us," he said, holding up the yucky brown bread.

I made a face. "But that one's ickier."

He laughed. "Only because your taste buds aren't used to it! Come on, we'll get some sandwich stuff and you'll adjust. And no more Miracle Whip; I think the second or third ingre-dient is high-fructose corn syrup. Mayonnaise is an awesome alternative; it's just a base of oil and eggs—we can even make it ourselves!"

The way Brady presented this was so simple that, over time, I became more and more interested in the relationship between our bodies and the foods we eat. What started with a comparison between two loaves of bread turned into a fas-cination with food, nutrition, and how it all worked together. After I had Avey, I recalled that conversation about the bread and started to reflect on my pregnancy and wonder how nu-trition might have affected the way it played out.

When I was pregnant with Avey, I knew that I needed to eat some kind of vegetables. I really loved salad, so I would grab one at Chick-fil-A or Wendy's, but my body would reject it every time. It didn't matter what kind of salad I tried—any fibrous vegetables and leafy greens I ate almost always came back up. I couldn't stand constantly throwing up, so I threw in the towel and primarily stuck to a French-fry-and-chicken-nugget diet throughout the pregnancy. Because I didn't realize the importance of proper nutrition at the time, it seemed like a fine diet to me. A bit further into the pregnancy, I broadened things a bit, adding some color to my diet—more specifically, the color orange. I would eat Cheetos for breakfast and homemade nachos for lunch. My favorite snacks were Preggie Pops, which are basically just candy. I'd eat them all day long. *Holy grams of sugar, Batman!*

I was a twenty-one-year-old woman with no nutritional background at all; I was clueless. Trying to grow and nourish the life of another human being while my body struggled to provide for its own led to disastrous results. Throughout my pregnancy with Avey, I believed I was healthy because all my blood work was within normal limits, but I never stopped to think about the facts *outside* of that blood work. From the time I was a child, I had an autoimmune disease that required daily medication. As I matured, I had wildly irregular periods; my hair wouldn't stop falling out; my nails were brittle and cracking; I had keratosis pilaris outbreaks that spread from my upper arms to my forearms, thighs, and bottom; I wore clinical-strength deodorant because I never stopped sweating, and my sweat would stain my clothing yellow, limiting the colors I was able to wear to mostly black. I had swelling issues in my extremities; I often developed mouth sores; I had major hand pain and was diagnosed with carpel tunnel syndrome. I had frequent headaches and migraines; I was constantly worried about plantar fasciitis because my dad had it and my feet were always in pain; and when I was in elementary school, I developed hemorrhoids. They became prolapsed in middle school due to bouts of constipation and compacted stool. By the time I was a teenager, the constant stress and strain on my anus caused anal fissures.

But despite the litany of medical issues I'd experienced, my hemoglobin, glucose, triglycerides, and cholesterol were all in the normal range during pregnancy, so in my mind, that meant I was healthy. At the time, I reasoned that my body's little quirks were just part of normal existence. None of it could be a direct reflection of the foods I was eating . . . right?

While I was nursing, one of the nicest things someone did for me was to wash a bunch of strawberries, blueberries, and pineapples and put them in a Tupperware bowl. Between nursing sessions, I could go to the fridge and eat fresh fruit quickly. I felt deeply cared for, and I realized it was an excellent example of how I should be caring for myself. I was beginning to recognize that I needed to get a handle on my eating; I just wasn't entirely sure how to do it. Over the years, I'd opted for highly restrictive diets, like going completely raw or plant-based, or multilevel-marketing programs that provided processed shakes, crappy supplements, and stimulants; I was overcomplicating something that in essence was very simple.

My desire to learn more inspired Brady and me to watch *Fat, Sick and Nearly Dead,* where Joe Cross saved his own life by juicing fruits, vegetables, nuts, and seeds. His auto-immune disease went into remission, and he also lost a tremendous amount of weight. That, for me, was eye-opening. I thought, *You're telling me that it could be as simple as eating real food? That this thing I've wrestled with my entire life might be healed by fruits and vegetables?* I had never thought about the possibility of improving the symptoms of my auto-immune disease. I was told by a doctor that I'd have to take pills for the rest of my life, and I'd accepted that; I'd never wondered if there might be another way. Then I thought about what the lactation consultants told me about Avey and breastfeeding—how it would be impossible. That memory sparked something in me. I realized that people in the medical profession might not have all the answers . . . and maybe it was time for me to take an active role in my own wellness to discover what those answers might be.

I realized that throughout my life, I'd put a lot of blame on other people. I now understood that lasting change could occur only when I acknowledged my own role in the situation. I had been complicit in my own decline, and knew I could no longer be a back-seat passenger in my own life. I began to understand that we need to eat the food that's already here on the planet, not the stuff that's made in a laboratory. God gave us everything we need to care for ourselves. To put this plan into action, Brady and I decided to buy a heavy-duty blender and a juicer. I was excited about juicing; I had learned that the pulp and fiber in fruits and vegetables help regulate the body's use of sugar, maintain the gastrointestinal lining, and provide prebiotic nourishment for beneficial gut bacteria. At the same time, juice is easier for the body to process and absorb; it provides instant energy, and it helps deliver as many nutrients as possible at one time. Instead of jumping into another difficult-to-maintain diet trend and focusing on how unfair it was that I had to avoid foods that aggravated my body, I worked on gradually adding positive steps to my daily routine.

For the first time in my life, I began to lose weight sustainably. I wasn't counting calories, and I wasn't being super-restrictive; I was just trying to be more mindful about the ingredients I was putting in my body. I still had the occasional slice of Costco pizza and chocolate froyo, but the way I viewed these things began to change. They became occasional treats rather than my main food source.

Instead of trying to eat perfectly, I focused on eating naturally, and I didn't beat myself up if I colored outside the lines every once in a while. I wasn't in a rush to shed the weight, though it was extremely gratifying to watch those numbers drop consistently and sustainably. Beyond losing weight, I placed value on taking care of myself because of the other benefits I began to experience.

My thought process was simple: If it comes from the earth, I'm going to eat it. I would juice for breakfast, eat a full meal for lunch, then have a light salad or smoothie for dinner. It wasn't always easy, but it was something that I could sustain. I learned that motivation is fleeting; it's something to be cherished when we have it, but maintaining any kind of lifestyle change is more about discipline and sticking to a schedule. I began to look at my eating as a chore, just another box on my daily to-do list that I needed to check off. This helped me overcome the roller-coaster diet cycle of starting something Monday, quitting it Thursday, bingeing over the weekend, then beginning a new regimen on Monday. The longer I sustained this mindset and method of eating, the more I enjoyed it. I went from being my mother's pickiest eater, with a diet that consisted mostly of "kid food"—Kraft mac and cheese, chicken fingers, and French fries—to someone who enjoyed eating brussels sprouts and salmon! Brady was right, taste buds do adjust. In fact, they don't just adjust, they regenerate—about every one to two weeks to be exact. This is great news for us picky eaters because it means that our bodies can develop a love for foods we once couldn't stomach.

Over the course of a year, I went from nearly 280 pounds to 190 pounds. Every time I went to see my physician, she lowered the dose of my thyroid medication, shocked at how drastically my numbers were improving. It was direct evidence that our bodies can regenerate, but what fuels regeneration? Whole foods. Our bodies are built on what we consume. The foods we eat can actually change our cellular structure. That's powerful stuff, man.

As I learned more, I started to grasp the full reality of our responsibility as parents. My choices as a mother directly affect my children, their perception, and their wellness. I didn't want to feed Avey the way my parents fed me—I wanted to give her the healthy food foundation I'd never had. I was determined that my children wouldn't have to endure the same struggles with obesity and chronic disease that I had. Subconsciously, I believed that saving them would be like having a do-over, enabling me to save myself. I was on fire for nutrition.

Every woman who has ever lost weight or found a diet that suits her perfectly knows what happens when those pounds begin to fall off—inevitably, something in her life or circumstances changes to radically shift her ability to maintain. For me, it was another pregnancy. During the early months of my pregnancy with our second child, I was terrified that something catastrophic would happen. All my doctors told me that what had happened with Avey was just a fluke. Even so, I was considered a high-risk pregnancy, which created a lot of anxiety for me. I found a new doctor, one who supported my desire to have a VBAC (vaginal birth after cesarean), and began to plan for another natural birth.

Though I'd been working on building a foundation of nutritional wellness, being pregnant caused me to return to a lot of old behavioral patterns. It was like muscle memory. When the going got tough and the pregnancy depleted my energy stores, I turned back to convenience foods; one enabled the other. I was too tired to prepare food, so I turned to fast or processed foods, but those foods held no nutritional value, further depleting my energy, which meant I had even less energy to cook real food. I ended up gaining fifty pounds. Although that's more than the recommended amount, it was still a big success for me because it was twenty pounds less than I'd gained during my pregnancy with Avey.

Again, I went into labor at thirty-nine weeks, and again I started working through it at home. Ultimately, I was in labor for forty-two hours, and never dilated past three centimeters.

The baby's head was stuck on the side of my pelvis and it was positioned sunny-side up. The doctors tried shifting its position and breaking my water, but twenty-four hours later, I still had no real progression, and my doctor told us it was time to call it and have another cesarean. I was so delirious from lack of sleep and pain, this time I gladly welcomed the surgery.

Our son Benjamin was a huge baby, a pure chunk—eight pounds, thirteen ounces. He made quite the entrance by peeing all over the doctor as soon as he came out (my kids love that story). The doctors told me his shoulders were so large that there was no way I could have birthed him vaginally without risking shoulder dystocia. This gave me a lot of peace about our decision to have a second cesarean.

Giving birth to Benjamin was an entirely different experience from having Avey. They held him up immediately; I was able to touch him over the sheet. My doctor told me they were going to take him to get cleaned up and weigh him, then they would bring him right back to me. I was so happy when they handed him over. I held him on my chest while they sewed me up. It was such a healing experience for me. They wheeled me into recovery with him still snuggled into me. I was able to put him on my breast right away. He took to breastfeeding like a duck to water; it was easy, like a match made in heaven—love at first sight. They never took him away from me again, and we lay skin to skin for hours.

During my pregnancy, my weight had climbed to 240 pounds, but I didn't moan over that. After all, I'd already unlocked the key to my own personal wellness. I'd lost the weight before, and I knew I could do it again. And I did. Through proper nutrition, by the time we reached Benjamin's first birthday, I'd gotten down to my lowest weight since high school—170 pounds—and was feeling confident in size 8 jeans.

I've always heard that it's hard going from one to two kids or from two to three. Going from one to two was seamless for me. Before Benjamin was born, I was worried that I wouldn't have enough love for both of them. Avey and I had become best friends and she was only eighteen months older than Benjamin. I didn't want her to feel neglected or as if she had been replaced. But when Benjamin was born, my love wasn't stretched thinner; my capacity for love literally grew. He fit in just fine with us, and because Avey was still in the baby phase, it didn't feel like I was adding more to my plate; it was just more of the same. I recovered quickly from my cesarean, as I had the first time, and we spent our days on the back porch, singing songs, making smoothies, and nursing on demand.

The summer after Benjamin turned one, Brady and I decided to visit my parents, who had moved back to California. Before we left, I told Brady that I was going to cut loose and eat whatever my little heart desired on our vacation. And that's exactly what I did. Anytime there was a pizza ordered, I sank my teeth into three or four delicious, cheesy slices. I ate tacos on the beach, drank milkshakes on the pier, and had buckets of French fries. After our trip ended and we were back in Texas, I was a little nervous about stepping on the scale. I knew that I had gained weight because all my clothes were tight and my size 8 jeans didn't fit anymore. Yet I had to know where I was if I wanted to get back to feeling good.

I wiggled my toes, stepped on the scale, and slowly looked down.

The needle was at 190 pounds.

I'd regained twenty pounds. I was shocked. I'd expected maybe ten . . . but twenty? Sure, I'd had a few splurges and a lot of tacos . . . but twenty pounds' worth? How could I have let this happen? I'd been doing so well and it felt like I'd just taken a giant leap backward. It didn't seem like a fair or even appropriate trade—twenty pounds for one week of eating a little bit extra? Did that mean that I could never splurge on vacation again? Why did my body hate me? Why did it hate food? Why couldn't I just be normal?

What I didn't realize then was that when you lose weight, it's easy to gain it back. The body's natural inclination is to store food for leaner times and get you back to your highest weight—it's a survival mechanism. Many people who struggle with morbid obesity are genetically inclined to gain weight easier or have fat-storage or hormonal disorders. It's why I could consume the same foods as my siblings or even eat less and gain weight while they maintained.

Many people don't realize that when they rapidly regain weight that it's not true weight gain. It's not necessarily fat adding pounds to the scale; it's inflammation or backed-up intestines or sodium and water retention. This is why it's crucial not to get discouraged and let a splurge meal, day, or week extend indefinitely. If you go back to mindfully eating, the pounds will fall off; it's when you let vacation follow you home that they start to stick around. Even though I didn't fully understand the science yet, I had a plan to get back to eating well after that first gain—

Then I found out that I was pregnant. Again.

20

Cardinals

Dear Body,
   I have felt abused by you, hurt by you in ways
that I've never been hurt by anything or anyone
else. Betrayed and then abandoned to deal with the
aftermath of things I felt were out of my control but
within yours. There were times when I didn't know if
I could ever forgive you.

While I was excited to discover I was pregnant again, I felt
I had been doing better with my health and dreaded gaining
all the weight back. But instead of getting lost in the worry, I
began to plan for a VBAC. I was still confident that my body
could birth a baby without a cesarean and I wanted to give
it every tool it needed to meet that goal. Because I'd had two
cesareans, in Texas it was no longer an option for me to try
for a vaginal delivery in a hospital, so I began interviewing
midwives for an out-of-hospital or birth-center birth.

Because of my risk factors—two cesareans, obesity, thyroid disease, IUGR (intrauterine growth restriction), placental abruptions, and now a baby with shoulders too wide to safely birth—it was not easy to find a midwife who would see me. But I knew that if Brady and I wanted to continue having children, I couldn't keep having cesareans. I'd already had two different OBs tell me that they limited their patients to three or four cesarean births. After that, they strongly recommended no more babies.

At this point in my life, my identity was entirely wrapped up in motherhood and being a wife. I was living my mom's dream of staying home and raising babies, I was fulfilling Brady's dream of working toward owning that secluded homestead, and accomplishing these things, at the time, felt like the fulfillment of my dreams as well.

I finally found two midwives who would take me on as a patient. Just days after making my decision on which practice I would go with and a week before our first prenatal appointment, while we were in the middle of a move into a house we were planning on renovating, I started bleeding. Just a little at first, then a little more, then a lot, accompanied by cramping. I was miscarrying. I didn't know how to feel about it. This pregnancy had been so brief, it was hardly like I was pregnant at all.

I felt bad because I didn't feel bad. I'd heard of women going through horrific miscarriages and suffering through their aftermath. But I was only around seven weeks pregnant at the time and miscarrying just felt like a delayed period. I struggled with not feeling sad, because I should have felt sad, right?

I rarely trusted my first emotional reaction to things, finding it strange that I didn't always respond the same way that others did. My closest female family members, my mother and my sister, had a wide breadth of emotional reactions, and mine never seemed to be as dynamic. I thought that this meant there was something wrong with me, like maybe I was broken. I did avoid certain emotions because I was afraid to feel them, but this wasn't that. I was just neutral toward my miscarriage, and I don't think that makes me a bad person. I think it makes me an honest one. Not everything that is sad feels sad, and that's okay.

Then before I knew it, I was pregnant again. Brady was working full-time and trying to do a complete remodel on the hundred-year-old house we'd moved into. There was no heat or air-conditioning. We had a jerry-rigged kitchen in one of the bedrooms that consisted of a hot plate and a countertop toaster oven. I began to battle extreme nausea again, this time while chasing after two toddlers, in a far from ideal situation.

My extended family complained about my living situation more than I did. But I was in my early twenties, and I always insisted, "It's not that bad, we're fine!" And at the time, that's what I really believed. But looking back at the seventy-year-old single-paned windows, moldy inner walls, and lack of climate control, I realize it really was bad.

Pregnancy and the ensuing nausea caused me to relapse once again into my old eating patterns—living off Sonic, Dairy Queen, and delivery pizza. As my due date approached, winter settled in. We were continuing to struggle to get by without heat. We had space heaters, but we couldn't have more than one plugged in at a time or we'd blow fuses in the old-school fuse box. We became a family who layered on hats, gloves, jackets, and three pairs of pants and spent the days snuggled under multiple blankets on the couch. It was too cold for me, so it would certainly be too cold for a newborn, although my toddlers seemed impervious to the cold.

With the biting cold of that winter pushing me over the

edge, I finally sat Brady down and said, "I can't do this any-more." While I was worried about the money we'd lose by abandoning our original plan, I'd already spoken with a real estate agent friend of mine and we figured out that we could sell the house without losing much more than what we'd put into it. I was ready to move forward with a new plan.

When Brady and I sat in that truck all those years ago talking about where we saw ourselves in ten years, Brady told me he wanted a forty-acre ranch with a creek and a pond. He wanted his own land to farm and his own animals to raise; he's always been on a quest for self-reliance. Every financial decision we made, in my mind, was an effort to get us closer to that dream of his. After a lengthy conversation, Brady agreed that it was time to cut our losses and sell both the duplex and the fixer-upper and finally invest in the dream.

That's when I found it.

I was doing what felt like an endless scroll, looking through properties on every site I could find. Then I came across a house in North Texas, near the Oklahoma border, that was interesting, but the description was confusing. The specs had it listed as three acres, but when I opened the map and looked more closely, I realized it wasn't three acres, but thirty-five—pretty darn close to the forty acres Brady had always wanted.

I immediately grabbed my phone and called the listing agent, who wasn't optimistic about the site. She let me know that it was an inherited property, owned by several siblings whose parents had passed away. Only one of the siblings was living there, and she was declining all showings. The real estate agent didn't think it was even worth trying to get a showing. I asked her what would happen if we just showed up. Was it illegal to knock on her door, introduce ourselves, and ask to see it? The agent laughed; she agreed that this was within our rights to do.

A few days later, Brady and I drove out to the house. I had Ben on my back, and Avey was standing between Brady and me, holding our hands, when we rang the bell. An older woman answered the door, and her eyes immediately lit up.

"I never have visitors," she said. "Please, come in, come in!"

The woman excitedly showed us around. The house needed work, but the property was a divine little slice of heaven; it was 40 percent heavily wooded, with two creeks and a pond. It also had an unfinished outdoor apartment that we could fix up and rent for extra income or use when friends and family came to stay with us. There were wild hogs and deer in the woods and plenty of space for goats and chickens. It was Brady's dream and I very much wanted to make Brady's dream come true.

We bonded with the woman over our Christian faith and listened to her stories about growing up on the property; she tearfully told us that the house was the only thing she had left of her father, who had built it himself. Finally, she said, "Okay, I'd like to sell the house. But I only want to sell it to you."

Brady was adamant there was no way we could ever swing it, but I knew we could. I could imagine us growing old there, raising our children, and rocking our grandbabies on the front porch. We were able to come up with the down payment and were thrilled that our little family was that much closer to living on Brady's near-perfect dream property (it was just missing those five acres).

The Lord has a funny way of working things out, because on the day of the closing, as we were signing the papers, our agent had a surprise for us. "Guess what? The property survey came back—it isn't thirty-five acres; it's forty," she said, rolling out the maps in front of us.

I squeezed Brady's hand and looked over at him as his face

pulled into a huge smile. It was like a little nod from the Lord that we were on the right path.

When we finally got the keys to the house, we felt such a mixed bag of emotions. At that point, I was two weeks away from giving birth—I was planning a home birth with a midwife—and we had to coordinate moving our young children and a houseful of stuff. Two days before moving day, the kids got a stomach bug the likes of which I'd never seen before and thankfully have not seen since. Brady and I were exhausted mentally and physically.

In the midst of all this, my mom called. Having moved back to California, she and my dad felt very far away during this time of extreme upheaval. After I had given her all the details of what was happening, she took a sharp inhale and said, "You can't handle this by yourself. I'm going to come there. I'll stay as long as you need me to." A mother always knows.

When my mom arrived just a few days later, I was so relieved. The day before, Brady and I had visited the property and were horrified by what greeted us—we had a mess on our hands. The previous owner had hired movers to come in and move her out, but anything she didn't want, she left in the house. All of the cupboards, the refrigerator, and the pantry were full of rotting food. There was stuff all throughout the house: clothing, trash, papers, piles of junk. The movers also hadn't worn foot covers and it had been snowing and pouring down rain, so in addition to the things left behind, the entire house was filled with leaves and dirt.

After surveying the property, Brady and I were speechless. There was not a single place, in the outdoor apartment or the house, that we could move our things into. It also dawned on me that I was in the midst of preparing for a tub birth at home, yet I didn't have a home to birth in. I started to cry;

my throat was tight, and I felt sick. There would be a baby in my arms the next week and I couldn't see a way we could get everything done in time, especially with the kids as sick as they were. I desperately tried to sort through the list of to-do items swirling in my head, but it seemed impossible. Just then, the baby kicked. I felt like it knew I was stressed and was supporting me from within. I took a breath, tried to relax, and rubbed my massive belly.

The next morning, my midwife reached out and said she wanted to come and check on me. Although I didn't want the midwife to see the house in this state, I was grateful she was coming by. She knew that I had begun to notice decreased fetal movement around thirty-two weeks, just like I had with Avey. But every health-care provider I talked to kept telling me it was my paranoia speaking. I'd gone to the ER two different times, at thirty-two weeks and thirty-six and a half weeks, to have a BPP (a biophysical profile—a nonstress test combined with ultrasounds) to ensure that everything was okay. Every time, the OBs told me everything was perfectly fine and that it was just my imagination, likely fueled by trauma. Even so, my instincts were screaming that something was wrong. But I had no medical evidence—just my intuition—and at that point, I didn't really trust my intuition when it came to my body. It had led me astray so many times.

That morning, Brady was out battling the deep snow and mud to get to town and buy supplies to fix a water line the movers had busted. My mom and the kids were still asleep. I had a few moments alone in the house for the first time. I walked around, trying to ignore all the dirt, grime, and stuff left behind, and stopped in the dining room to look out the window onto the blanket of snow that covered everything in sight. The light bouncing off the snow was perfect, creating an ethereal glow in the house that illuminated dancing dust. As I looked over the yard, a cardinal landed right in front of the window.

I smiled.

Then another cardinal landed.

My smile widened.

Then another landed, and another, and another, until there were about twenty brilliant red cardinals on the snow. My mom came to look and so did the kids; we all marveled at the sight. It was as if they were there just for us.

We were so enthralled, I jumped when my midwife knocked on the door. She walked in and I immediately relaxed into her familiar warmth. As we sat on the dining-room floor and chatted about preparations, she looked over and noticed the cardinals dancing in the snow and said, "That's the most extraordinary thing I've ever seen. I've never seen so many cardinals in one place."

After that, we went through my birth plan. She told me she had the inflatable tub in her car and that we'd set it up right there in the dining room. Then she suggested we check on the baby one more time. Avey ran in as soon as she saw the Doppler come out, and she and my midwife knelt by my side. Avey began to glide the Doppler over my belly, and my mom thought it was the cutest thing and started snapping pictures.

My mom and I continued chatting as Avey ran the Doppler all over my belly. Soon, the midwife said, "Hey, Avey, let me see that for a minute."

That's weird, I thought. It was taking a really long time, but I was still only half paying attention as the midwife pushed the Doppler harder into my sides. I noticed my mom's expression slowly begin to change.

Finally, my midwife stopped completely, folded the Doppler up, put it down, and leaned over to me. Her eyes were shining with tears as she said, "We need to go to the hospital right now."

"Is everything okay?" I asked. "Are we okay?"

"Yep, we're fine," she replied. "Let's just go to the hospital now."

"Should I get my bag?"

"No, let's just go."

As the midwife helped me up, Brady walked into the room. My mom stayed behind with the kids, and Brady and I hopped in the car. We drove to the closest hospital, but they didn't have a labor and delivery department, so we had to turn around and drive all the way in the opposite direction. We were in the car for an hour and a half; the whole time I was feeling my stomach and saying to Brady:

"I'm sure I feel the baby."

"I'm sure I felt movement."

"I don't remember it really moving a ton last night, but babies get bigger and their movements change."

"Okay, I did just feel it move."

"It moved, it moved, it moved."

"It's fine, everything's fine."

I was just talking, a stream of questions and reassurances spoken to myself, to Brady, to the baby. The entire time, Brady tried to gently ask exactly what had happened, but I didn't have any answers to give.

The midwife had already called ahead, so when we arrived at the hospital, we were taken straight up to labor and delivery. They got me on a monitor right away, and the nurse said, "Okay, okay, there's a heartbeat."

"See? Yeah," I said, relaxing. "Everything's fine. I was sure I felt the baby moving when we were on the way here."

"Yes, there's a heartbeat," she said. "It's a little bit fast to be your heart, so I'm thinking this should be the baby, but we're going to get the ultrasound tech in here and we'll figure it all out. I'm sure everything's fine."

"Great, thank you." I took a deep breath and sank into the bed.

The ultrasound tech came in and set the ultrasound wand on my tummy. I stared at the screen. And then I saw it, the place on the monitor that should show the heartbeat. The line was flat.

Someone took a gulping breath of air.

I looked at Brady and he was crying.

I'd never seen him cry before.

But then I was crying too.

My mom was unable to come with the kids because of the snow, so Brady and I journeyed through the nightmare alone, together. Others offered to come but I didn't want to see anyone. There wasn't a chapter about this in any of the baby books we'd read; this was uncharted territory. We had to wait several hours because the doctor who would perform the C-section was delivering another baby. A social worker came in, handed us a list of funeral homes, and instructed us to pick one to send the body to.

Finally, I was wheeled into the operating room and the C-section began. Tears ran down my face as they cut into me and I felt the familiar sensation of pressure and pulling. I tried to send my mind far away. I didn't want to know this kind of pain.

Everything after that was a blur. I was wheeled into a recovery room and they soon brought the baby boy we'd agreed to name Elias in for us to see. They had him bundled up in a blanket with a hat on. I wanted to unwrap him so I could see all his little parts. They agreed to unwrap him just enough so I could see his little feet and hands. We only had minutes with him because the funeral home had shown up to take his body away, and it was getting late and they were about to close.

Being in that hospital room that night brought me back to Avey's birth—how they had taken her away and I was in my room feeling like I'd never had a baby at all. I was experiencing the same kind of feeling, but tinged with a deep, hollow sadness I'd never felt before. I'd just had a baby, the wounds were still raw, but now I was an empty vessel and my baby wasn't somewhere within the hospital walls being fed and kept warm. He was gone.

Forever.

Finally, I drifted off to sleep, haunted by the sounds of babies crying in the rooms next door.

As I came back into consciousness, the pain returned, as did my debilitating grief. The door creaked open, and a nurse walked in. As she took my vitals, she looked at me with pity in her eyes and said, "I'm so sorry this happened to you. My sister had a miscarriage last year and it was just so hard on her—on the whole family, really."

"I'm so sorry for your loss," I whispered.

"I really feel for you; it was so hard on all of us," she said before making a few notes in my chart and leaving.

Tears spilled from my eyes. I never wanted anyone to say anything like that to me again. There was no possible way this person—distant from a loss that was completely different from the one I'd just experienced—could ever understand my pain. Yet she was, by no means, the last person to attempt to comfort me with words like that.

When I look back on the times that I've felt true, bone-crushing grief, like I did after we lost Elias, I realize that silence—the gap created by loss—can be too much for some people to bear. Often, they attempt to fill that space with words. Those words are meant to extend a hand, some measure of understanding, some way to relate. Everyone means well, but attempts at antidotal condolences like "It's okay because he's in heaven now" or "This was all part of God's plan" or "At least you still have Avey and Ben" did little to help or comfort or soothe the gaping, empty hole that seemed to have appeared overnight and that I began to let myself fall into.

21

Aftermath

Dear Body,
*   I never knew that pain that wasn't physical could*
be quite so overwhelming. Losing a child is the
greatest source of pain I've ever known. And because
I felt responsible, because I believed that I was the
cause, it became my greatest source of shame.

All I wanted to do after losing Elias was leave the hospital. The constant sound of joy-filled voices in the hallway and tiny baby cries from the rooms surrounding mine made me feel like I was losing it. It was as if I was being haunted by what could have been. In larger hospitals, they have a bereavement wing, far away from the sounds of families celebrating and welcoming new life. But our hospital was small, and the labor and delivery and postpartum units were combined into one. I was surrounded by the sounds of women giving birth, newborn cries, and big congratulatory families and the fanfare that usually accompanies such a momentous occasion.

I begged Brady to take me home. He and I fought with the nursing staff to release me early from the hospital. Because I'd had a cesarean, I was supposed to stay at least forty-eight hours.

After we spoke with the doctor, she agreed to release us after twenty-four hours, as long as we promised that we would return if I began to show signs of infection. We left, but we couldn't go home yet. We had one harrowing stop to make. The funeral home had asked us to come by as soon as possible so we could make arrangements for Elias's body. Our parents and my grandparents met us at the funeral home. We had been told that we would be able to see and hold Elias, but when we arrived, they said his little body shouldn't be viewed again. I remember feeling so bad because I'd told my mom not to come to the hospital, that she would get to see him at the funeral home, and now she'd never get to see him. Brady and I would forever be the only ones who had seen his face, held his hand, kissed his head. I felt like I'd robbed my family of their chance to know him too.

In the lobby of the funeral home, my grandpa wrapped me in his arms, and I cried. I just kept doing that. Crying. All the time. And when I wasn't crying, I felt like people were judging me, thinking, *Shouldn't she be crying?*

I hated crying. It made me feel embarrassed and vulnerable, naked in a way I never wanted to be in front of other people. They could have my joy; I was all too happy to share sunlight and radiant blissful moments with others, but this? I didn't want to share this. It was hard and sad and I didn't even know how to navigate the treacherous cliffs of grief and devastation myself, let alone how to shepherd anyone else through it. I didn't want to be subjected to their thoughts and condolences. I knew they were trying to make me feel loved, but instead they made me feel suffocated. I wanted to retreat.

As we headed to the car, I told my mom I didn't want to be alone but that I wanted to be selective about who I had around me. As someone who learned to bury emotions at an early age, I was scared to feel those big, all-consuming feelings. I didn't know how to hold them, work through them. I didn't even trust that I was actually feeling them correctly. I needed space to work it all out. I told my mom that the only people I wanted around were her, Brady, and Aunt Kim. I knew that I needed to protect my peace, and Mom, Brady, and Aunt Kim were my peacekeepers.

When we pulled into the driveway of our new dream home, my chest felt tight. I dreaded walking into the house with the messy rooms, the musty smell, the mattress on the floor. As I stared at the door, all I could see was my midwife's tearful eyes as she told me, "We need to go to the hospital." I already knew what I would discover when we walked inside, what I would feel. I wanted to find another home; this one already held ghosts.

Brady opened the car door and guided me to the house because I was still unable to walk upright or unassisted yet. Then he opened the front door, and I walked over the threshold. I could hardly believe my eyes. The whole living room was set up—our furniture was there, all arranged, and a candle burned on the mantel. I walked through the house and saw that all of our belongings had been moved in. The master bedroom was set up, the kids' beds were made, the kitchen was clean and stocked with fresh food. The carpets had been shampooed; the bathrooms deep-cleaned.

I looked at my mom, tears tracking down my cheeks again. "You did this?"

She smiled. "We all did."

Everybody in our life had shown up to help ready our home for our arrival—church friends, my grandparents, my aunt Kim, family friends Georgia, Selena, and Kelley. They brought husbands, sons, and other male relatives to move the furniture while the women got on their hands and knees and scrubbed that beat-up old house until it shone. My mom organized it all. They'd set up the rooms so that I would have a nice home to come back to. They'd hid all of the baby stuff so I didn't have to see it. In the midst of one of the worst moments of my life, it was like the entire world was saying, *We love you and we're going to get you through this.*

And they said it without words.

As time went on, I started to settle into my new normal as a grieving mother. When you experience a major trauma, the world watches you more closely, treats you more cautiously, and acts like you should be kept under glass, untouched. Although I appreciated the concern, there were some people who just didn't know how to handle those in mourning. Everything penetrates more deeply when you're grieving. Words I could have easily dismissed before stuck with me, got under my skin, and made me angry. And it was a relief to feel angry, because it offered a break from being sad. With Elias's death, it seemed my whole universe had gone sad, and I was supposed to present myself to the world as sad from that moment forward. But grief isn't just sadness; it's multifaceted. It's many different things at once.

Early on, in the hospital, I'd started to learn that so much of dealing with grief is about handling the way others react to your pain. That's why I stayed secluded for a while. I just didn't want to have anybody else's interpretations floating around, further complicating things. Sometimes, however, I'd make exceptions for family. Not long after we lost Elias, one of my aunts came over. She sat across from me, leaned forward with her elbows propped on her knees, and asked, "Have you even cried yet?"

I couldn't formulate a response. I can only imagine the look on my face as I thought, *Are you kidding me?*

Heaven forbid I don't cry in front of every person I know. That certainly means I don't care, right?

Or maybe I just don't want to cry in front of certain people, so I choke back tears?

Maybe I feel nothing?

Maybe I feel too much?

Maybe I feel angry?

Maybe I've just run out of frickin' tears.

That's the thing about grief. It doesn't always look the way people expect it to. It's not always screaming, sobbing, wailing, and ripping clothes. Sometimes it looks like quiet reflection. Sometimes it looks like crying in the shower so you don't scare your toddlers. Sometimes it looks like abandoning your cart and leaving Target empty-handed because there were just too many pregnant bellies around. Sometimes it looks like nothing at all.

But it's always there. Because it's love trapped inside you with no place to go.

At first grief was loud, then it was quiet, and now it's something I live with every day. It's mine to carry till heaven, when I finally get to embrace my child again. There are moments—even as I write this now—that it roars and rages and I remember the injustice of it all. But mostly, it sits quietly, always there, like an Elias-shaped hole in the center of my soul.

A week after I had Elias, my mom scheduled her flight to go back home. She had been helping us the whole time, cooking dinner, watching the kids, and cleaning the house. On top of organizing moving and cleaning crews, she started a meal train to keep us fed and our pantry stocked. I can't even imagine what going through that time would have been like without my mom.

On the last day she was with us she suggested, "Why don't you and Brady go out for lunch or something and I'll watch the kids? It's the last chance you'll have to take advantage of a free babysitter for a while."

Brady and I took her up on it and we went to shower and get ready. In those early days, I really didn't like the shower. I could busy myself all day with chores, tasks, and kids, but as soon as I stepped into that little box, I was alone. My thoughts could assault me without distraction. And I had some pretty volatile thoughts. I stood there with the hot water pouring over my body. My breasts were tender and engorged because my milk had come in, but I had no child to feed. My belly still looked pregnant.

I began to pray. I asked the Lord *why*. I lamented that He hadn't taken me too. I told Him that if this was His plan, I didn't know if I wanted to be a part of it anymore.

In that moment, words filled my spirit. I've never heard the audible voice of the Lord, but if you believe in the Holy Spirit, you'll know what I mean when I say that His word can descend on your spirit in an instant and you just *know* that it's divine and that it's *Him*. For the first time since Elias was born, I felt peace; I felt understanding. I felt God.

And I felt like I knew why we'd lost him.

I carefully stepped out of the shower, put clothes on slowly to avoid touching my C-section incision, then got into the car with Brady. As I pulled on my seat belt, he looked over at me and said, "The craziest thing happened when I was in the shower. The Lord told me something."

Letting my seat belt retract back, I turned to face Brady. "Me too," I whispered reverently.

"He said that He took him now because we were going to lose him later—"

I gasped and cut him off. "Yes, he was going to be taken from us in a terrible way that we wouldn't be able to heal from."

Brady nodded as his eyes watered.

"I felt like He said that we wouldn't be able to make it through that loss. I felt like He knew that we could bear it now—this way." I sniffed.

Brady grabbed hold of my hand tightly and we thanked the Lord for helping us understand.

Just then, a red cardinal landed on the tree in front of us, and I knew that we were going to be okay.

22

Trophies

Dear Body,
    From the earliest moments of my life, I knew that
I would be a mother. I imagined myself barefoot in a
sundress standing on a front porch, my arms wrapped
around my swollen belly and the wind in my hair. But
in all of my wildest imaginings, never did I think that
my body, created to hold life, would give me death.

One bright light during this time was our new home. It did
us all good to be surrounded by forest, wildlife, and towering
trees, far outside the city and away from everyone. We were
isolated, but that was perfect for me. I didn't want to see other
people anyway.

The property was the manifestation of everything Brady
had told me he ever wanted. I had wholeheartedly believed
that moving to the ranch—achieving this part of the plan we
had for our lives—would make Brady happier than he'd ever

been. But that just didn't happen, and that was adding to the weight of my already unbearable grief.

As the oldest in a large family, I often felt responsible for peacekeeping. I had to ensure that everyone stayed calm and happy. I had to entertain my siblings, make sure they had everything they needed. I had to please my parents, make sure they stayed even-keeled and in bright spirits. I wore their expectations and happiness on my shoulders, like trophies on a mantel. It was only natural that, after I got married, I would feel responsible for Brady's happiness as well. I didn't even realize I was doing it. I couldn't bear the thought of him being unhappy. But it seemed like there was always something keeping him from true happiness, and I subconsciously felt that if I just worked hard enough, I could obtain it for him.

When we first found the house, I envisioned him waking up early and heading out to his workshop with a hot cup of tea, spending the morning turning pieces of wood into furniture, then coming back in to grab the kids to work in the garden before venturing into the woods for a bit of afternoon adventure. Yet nothing seemed to change for Brady. If anything, getting his dream property only seemed to make him less happy. He was busy with work, and when he was home, there was always a lot going on with the kids or something that needed fixing in the house, shop, or yard, so he wasn't able to devote himself to the things he'd imagined he'd be doing. He has always been his own harshest critic, as most of us are. Most of his unhappiness came from within, things within himself he was displeased with. Although his mood was less of a reflection on me and what I wasn't bringing to the table, our married life certainly wasn't the glamorized version we had both pictured.

Our expectations of each other were not aligning. I'd been

pregnant our entire marriage. For four straight years, I'd been couch-ridden, bedridden, dealing with all-day sickness, or breastfeeding. I was always behind on household duties, and at that point, I wasn't even able to take good care of myself. They say that in marriage it isn't fifty-fifty but one hundred–one hundred, and for those years Brady was having to give one hundred and fifty to my fifty, with little reprieve. He understood, and it wasn't that life was bad or that we weren't getting along. We were surviving. But we wanted to thrive.

We did silly things to make sure we prioritized each other. The problem was, although we were making time for each other, we weren't really connecting during that time. There was so much we weren't talking about or that we avoided talking about because it was uncomfortable. I didn't want to hear his displeasure with the way that I was keeping up with my duties because I already felt like I was carrying too much. I also didn't want to face some of the things in our marriage that *I* was personally dissatisfied with.

On top of that, Brady and I were working through our grief in different ways. We didn't talk to each other much about it. He would try to listen, but when I'm emotional, I tend to just talk and talk and talk. I remember one time, I was talking to Brady in bed, starting to really open up to him about how I felt about Elias. I came to a natural break in my monologue and Brady didn't say anything. I wiped tears from my eyes, looked over, and saw he was fast asleep.

Despite all this, as Brady and I traversed life together, we maintained our strong bond. I never faltered for a moment in my love for him, and I considered him not only my husband but my best friend. Tumultuous times will do that to a couple. They'll shake things up; they'll cause chaos; they'll force you to find new ways to love and support each other even if, often, they create distance.

I was focused wholly on getting through each day. I was taking care of Avey and Ben, keeping up with the laundry, and trying to make our new house a home. I rarely wore anything other than one of the printed oversize sleep T-shirts my mom bought me after I delivered. I stopped showering. Makeup was a thing of the past; most days I couldn't even be bothered to brush my hair.

When I did have to get dressed to go out, I would spend the entire time telling Brady how much I hated my body—how it looked, how it felt, how it wasn't fair for it to be postpartum. Nothing fit, and I refused to wear the maternity clothes that had so recently cradled my growing belly and were now filled with memories of nothingness. I couldn't articulate how betrayed I felt. It was as though I were a stranger in my own body; I had no snuggly baby to get me through the awkward stage my body was in and no way to explain my situation to strangers who still asked with beaming smiles, "When are you due?"

I spent most days in bed. We used to have strict screen-time regulations for the kids, but it was easier for me to let *Mickey Mouse Clubhouse* play while I tried to sleep, all three of us curled up together. I avoided my phone and the constant text messages that all asked the same thing: How are you?

How am I?

How do you think I am?

I want to die.

Then I'd remember the response I'd trained myself to give and would type back, *Fine!* ☺

But I wasn't fine. I was drowning in a sea of grief without any idea how to swim. No one had ever taught me how to swim through it. Were we just supposed to know? Was this a trial I was just thrown into and that I was supposed to figure out on my own? It was ingrained in me to present to people the person they wanted to see instead of who I actually was. So I performed expertly and people praised how well I was doing and how strong I was, even though I wasn't well or strong at all.

I was avoiding.

I was self-medicating with food.

I was burying, burying, burying—with television, binge-fests, house projects, and feigned happiness.

My midwife recommended I attend a grieving mothers' group, but I didn't want to leave the house and felt like it would just make me sadder. I didn't want to have to listen to everyone else's dead-baby stories. How could that be healing for me? Sometimes, though, real joy would sneak in, peeking through the clouds for fleeting moments. Joy was an emotion that confused me. In those moments I wondered how I could be both happy and sad. The joy of having toddlers who learned new things every day, said silly things, and splashed through the puddles when it rained would make me laugh and then I would immediately reprimand myself, thinking, *How could you be laughing after all you've been through? After what you've lost?*

Despite the guilt, I would hold on to joy whenever I could find it. I'd stash it away, store it up, and use it when I needed it most, like toxic positivity. I used any morsel of joy I could muster to try to bury the undercurrent of mourning, but it wasn't an effective burial. It was as though I'd placed it all in a shallow grave; the grief kept bubbling to the surface, and I couldn't figure out how to get it to stop. I just knew that I didn't want to surrender myself to it. I was already so broken, I feared that if I let myself truly feel it all, I'd never be able to come back from it.

Life marches forward, though. I felt stuck in this horrible place, but the rest of the world just went on. The kids continued to grow, the weeks passed quickly, and we began to talk about me getting pregnant again. Would we prevent it? Should I go on birth control? Because I wasn't breastfeeding and my milk had dried up about a month after I gave birth, we knew I would probably begin to ovulate again soon. Benjamin was nearing three; Brady and I both felt like we wanted to have one more baby and then put the childbearing years behind us. Neither of us wanted a large age gap between the kids, so we decided not to prevent pregnancy. Some friends and family were surprised that we didn't opt for preventive measures, but my body had been pregnant for the past year and a half with no newborn to show for it. It felt like a wrong I needed to right. Not to replace Elias, of course—I could never—but I knew that experiencing a live birth again would bring healing to my soul.

Part of the trade that you make during pregnancy is sacrificing your body for a child. But when you sacrifice your body and you don't get a child—I don't know that I can adequately put into words how wrong it feels. It felt wrong to have breast milk but no babe to feed, to have a soft, squishy postpartum belly but no newborn to snuggle. It felt wrong to recover from yet another cesarean birth without being able to lie and stare at a new little life.

Two months after we had Elias, I got pregnant. I was cautiously optimistic but already starting to feel the toll the anxiety of the unknown would take on me during another pregnancy.

At nine weeks, I miscarried again.

My second miscarriage was more difficult than the first and I began to wonder if my body was even capable of carrying another healthy pregnancy to term. I began to wonder what the hell I was doing that was so wrong. I was young, and my mom had had seven pregnancies back to back and she'd never had these issues. I felt like my body had betrayed me.

I felt like it was actively working against me, and I couldn't figure out why.

I don't know exactly how much I weighed at that time. Losing weight was the last thing on my mind. I was probably close to two hundred and fifty pounds. Any apprehension I had over entering a new pregnancy before losing the postpartum weight was overshadowed by my need to restore and heal. When we received Elias's autopsy and pathology report, we realized the complications he'd experienced were a carbon copy of what had happened with Avey: IUGR, placental abruption (times two), and insufficient placental function.

Finding this out made me so angry because I *knew*.

I'd told my midwife, my doctor, and the physicians in the ER that something wasn't right. I'd said the words over and over: "I think he has IUGR just like Avey."

They always responded, "He doesn't. There is nothing on his scans to confirm that."

And then I'd say, "Well, you didn't see it on hers either."

I pushed for more testing. I'd had two level-two sonograms, countless nonstress tests and biophysical profiles, appointments just for monitoring, and several emergency trips to the ER . . . because I knew.

I just knew.

And then I found out I was pregnant again.

When you're pregnant, it's natural to begin to dream, dream about what life will be like when that new little being joins your world. *What will it look like? Will it be a boy or a girl? Let's get a nursery together; what should the theme be?* But I wouldn't allow myself to dream this time, because with the possibility of a live baby came the possibility of a dead baby, and I was still haunted by dreams of the doctor holding Elias over that sheet, his little, lifeless body just flopping over. I was convinced that this baby would greet me that way too.

It felt like I had been pregnant for so long at that point. I was anxious and paranoid. I was constantly going to the ER to get checked out. Sometimes I spent entire days and nights attached to a monitor. But the medical staff was gracious. They understood.

I was scheduled for a cesarean in mid-April. It's standard practice: If you have fetal demise after thirty-eight weeks, they can schedule your next birth at thirty-eight weeks. If I could have scheduled it even sooner, I would have. Honestly, I felt like the safest place for the baby growing in my belly was on the outside where capable hands could reach over and help.

After having two babies with placental ruptures and IUGR, I found an ob-gyn who specialized in high-risk pregnancies. He said I was presenting with classic signs of a blood-clotting disorder, though all of my lab work was negative. Regardless, he said that the blood can't tell you everything and he decided to treat me like a patient with a blood-clotting disorder. I went in weekly for B_{12} and blood-thinner injections; I was put on baby aspirin and a prescription prenatal vitamin with methylfolate instead of folic acid, which he referred to as "dangerous garbage."

I no longer had any desire to try to have a vaginal birth, finally getting the picture that my body just really, really didn't want to do that. It also felt far less important now. All I could think about was making it to April.

23

Betrayal

Dear Body,
   When you're betrayed by a lover, it's not just
a sin against your heart and soul; it's a sin against
your body as well. Some may blame themselves and
pit the soul against the body, wondering what they
could have done differently. But that is often just
a distraction from the root of the issue: the lack of
communication and honesty between you and your
partner. A trespass in a physical relationship with a
partner is a trespass against the whole.

When I was eight months pregnant with Noah, dealing with anxiety on a level that I have never experienced before, just a month after our five-year wedding anniversary, I discovered something that Brady had hidden from me. It was a marital betrayal the likes of which our marriage had never experienced. It was not an affair, but it felt to me like it might as well have been one.

I've gone over and over this in my mind; I've consulted with other writers, editors, and Brady on what to share and how much to share so I could convey the depth of the harm and the betrayal but also preserve the relationships of those involved. For those who know me, I am an open book. If we were sitting down with each other face-to-face, discussing our deepest secrets in confidence, I wouldn't hesitate to share every detail with you.

But this book will be published for the world to see, and not all people are kind, forgiving, and understanding, especially regarding situations they've never been through themselves. The written word also leaves things to interpretation, and while I feel strongly that this story is one I need to share, I also feel I must do so without providing every detail. Brady has given me his permission and his blessing to share whatever I want to—he says that he deserves every unkind word and thought someone might utter or think—but I don't want to completely open him or me up to others' judgment. His betrayal was a trespass against our relationship, and we healed from it and moved past it years ago.

It's important to me that I share this story because it's easy to look at a couple's highlight reel on social media and believe that they have a perfect relationship and that everything they do is #couplegoals. It's easy to think that maybe there's something wrong with you because your relationship is a little messier than that. It's not all pin-worthy romantic getaways, extravagant gifts, or sweet little thoughtful gestures done "just because." All of us have skeletons in our closets, things we've gone through, cried through, felt we'd be torn apart over.

I've learned that there are parts of marriage that should be kept quiet to both protect each other and preserve the respect and the sanctity of the relationship. You may confide many things to your very best friend about your spouse, but there are parts that are truly meant for you two alone, because no one is going to love you and know all of the ins and outs of you like that other person does. A partner has the ability to see you in a multidimensional, stripped-down, worst and best kind of way and accept you because of and in spite of it. The world doesn't love you like that, though. Most people have no commitment to you. And I've learned that if there's something they can use against you, they will. This is not an encouragement to keep quiet about domestic abuse or to stay in a relationship that is hurting you; it's just an explanation why I, and most of us, don't share everything on the worldwide stage.

The year 2016 was indescribably difficult for me. I was reliving pregnancy trauma, scared out of my mind that my body would not be able to support another pregnancy, battling grief, still not even a year postpartum, and struggling to keep my head above water. I was drowning, but instead of calling for help, I pretended to swim. I escaped into reality TV, and Brady escaped into video games, and if anyone had asked, I would have said that we were happy. But looking back, I don't think that we were happy; I think that we just weren't fighting.

With the distance between us and everything we were dealing with, some might not find it a shock if one or both of us got caught up in something extramarital. But I was filled with so much unbelief when confronted with the truth that my mind literally made up excuses to justify what I'd found. When I asked him, it was innocent, not accusatory; I actually laughed and joked as I tossed out scenarios that I was sure had nothing to do with Brady because they couldn't have had anything to do with Brady. It was completely out of character for him. I know there will be friends and family who will read these words and won't be able to believe them. Because Brady is one of the good ones; truly, down to his bones, he is so good. But his pain and the stress of the past few years manifested differently for him than it did for me.

He stopped me quickly and sat down on the bed like something indiscernibly heavy was on his shoulders. He came out with the truth immediately, didn't try to make excuses or hide it. He apologized over and over, and all I remember feeling was nothing. I think I was in shock, because if there was anyone I trusted not to hurt me, it was him. And this was definitely the worst way that a partner could have hurt me. It wasn't the actual deed but what it represented—that I didn't know this person as well as I thought I did. He was someone who suddenly was capable of secrecy and trespass. And, of course, it was the betrayal.

I demanded answers, which he supplied abundantly. He said that he'd wanted to tell me for so long, but he was afraid that I would leave him when what he really needed was for me to help him. He said he felt relieved that I finally knew, no matter what choice I made, to stay or not to stay.

That night, for the first time in our marriage, I made him sleep somewhere else. It's not often that I don't have words, but I truly didn't have any words. I felt like his presence alone was keeping me from rational thought. We had children to consider—I was getting ready to deliver another in just a few more weeks—so I knew that I needed to navigate this situation very carefully. I needed to protect myself and do what was in my best interests but also theirs. I just wasn't quite sure what that was.

Usually, I would grab the phone and call Aunt Kim, talk out all of my stuffed-up feelings with her. But I knew that even though she loved us both, she loved me first and best; he would be judged, and harshly. Even though I was angry with him and deeply hurt, I still wanted to protect him. Because I know that we're more than the sum of our worst deeds.

The next day, I called his sister. I needed to unburden myself and I knew that I could tell her he'd committed murder and she'd still meet him with love. She was as speechless as I was. She offered prayer and continued moral support, and I felt better just having someone to talk to, even though the waters were muddied, and I felt completely unprepared to handle something of this magnitude.

After Brady arrived home that evening and we'd put the kids to bed, we sat down in the living room to talk. I wish I could say I maintained a cool head, but I didn't; I raged, I cried. I also bemoaned the fact that if I decided to leave, I had nothing—no education, no job, no money—and I had two children to take care of and was pregnant with a third. Meanwhile, he would be fine. He'd continue in his career, see his kids on the weekend, and be no less attractive to prospective partners. He'd find a new woman, create a new family, and cut me a child-support check, which probably wouldn't cover even a quarter of our expenses, even though I had worked just as hard as he had. I had sacrificed my whole life to build his dreams.

We might heal, we might make it through this, but I made a promise to myself at that moment: Never again would I be this dependent on anyone. Fool me once and all that. He understood; he agreed; he was sorry. I told him that I hadn't decided what I was going to do yet but if we stood any chance, he needed to figure out how to make it right on his own. I wasn't going to instruct him; I was his wife, not his mother. This was his mess, and while I loved him enough to let him try, I wasn't going to fix it for him.

He began attending counseling and a men's group at church,

completely unprompted by me. He asked me if I would be his accountability partner. We had heard a message in church about the brain and how it forms patterns of thought. The average person has five hundred unwanted thoughts a day that are about thirteen seconds in length. That means that two hours of every day is spent on unwanted thoughts. The way you think changes the way that you behave because life is always moving in the direction of your strongest thoughts. And the more you dwell on something, the stronger the pattern it creates in your mind.

The pastor used an illustration that I thought was very powerful. He told us about his mother's front yard, how she'd spent years landscaping it perfectly. She had beautiful grass, perfectly trimmed hedges, flowers planted just right, and clearly marked paths so that everything stayed pristine. One day, she got a new mailman, and instead of taking the marked path, he walked through her grass. He did this day after day, week after week, until suddenly her grass was no longer pristine but had a clearly marked trench the mailman had worn. It wasn't long after this that the pastor showed up at his mother's home to find her paving a new walkway. When he asked her what she was doing, she said, "If he's going to walk it anyway, I might as well make it look nice."

The pastor's point was that some of us are so rehearsed in sin that we have paved the pathway for it. We have to rehearse the truth more than we rehearse the lie, the pain, the trauma, the addiction. We can't forge new paths by continuing to walk the ones that haven't been serving us.

Confiding in a friend, diverting the thought pattern, and telling yourself the truth are the pillars to begin abandoning the old paths and creating the new. I agreed to be Brady's accountability partner. In doing so, I was acknowledging that it wasn't me versus him but us against the problem. I agreed to listen with an open mind and heart and not let my emotions get in the way of what we were striving toward, which was healing. It's important to note that I still loved him very much. I was angry, hurt, betrayed, and confused, but I'd married him for a reason. Every part of me loved him and wanted to see this through with him, just not at the expense of my or my children's well-being.

Healing from this kind of betrayal and moving forward as a couple works only if you're both in it. Even after receiving confirmation that he was, I had to give myself space and time to discover if *I* was. The person who was supposed to love me the most had betrayed me. I'd also begun to discover how multidimensional we all are. After having lost a child, I was able to hold both grief and joy in my heart simultaneously. I figured that this form of betrayal was just like that grief, and if I could hold joy alongside the grief, maybe I could still hold love too.

And yet thoughts began to invade my mind: that Brady really wanted to be with someone else, that the real reason he wasn't happy was because he wasn't happy with me, and that anyone would be a better wife to him than me. If I were skinny, would this have happened? If I had been better at keeping house and managing all of my homemaker duties, would he still have done it? Was there some kind of failure to be, do, or act on my part that had brought this piece of him to the surface?

I began to convince myself that he didn't really love me, even though all of his actions were telling me the opposite. He was doing the work, not just for himself and not just in counseling. We would go through homework that he'd assigned himself. His actions were bringing us closer together, but in the state I was in—pregnant and scared, lonely and grieving, betrayed and so sad—it was easier to let my worst insecurities and fears take hold.

I rehearsed this way of thinking and I saw a shift in my extroverted nature. I had already become more reclusive, but after Brady's misstep, I withdrew from the world around me. I drew away from my closest friends, finding it easier not to pick up the phone than to talk while keeping the biggest part of my life a secret.

Even though Brady was doing the work, even though we were getting better, I was falling apart in a new way. Brady's choices had opened a Pandora's box in my mind. Something I'd never thought was possible had happened; what else that I'd thought wasn't possible could?

24

Rainbow

Dear Body,

You can hold so many things within you at once: sadness, grief, anger, love, joy, and happiness; they all exist alongside one another. Even during seasons of tremendous turmoil and pain, we are not given over to only those experiences but also to ones that provide relief. As Stephen Chbosky says in *The Perks of Being a Wallflower*, "So, this is my life. And I want you to know that I am both happy and sad and I'm still trying to figure out how that could be." It resonates because it's true; sometimes I am happier, sometimes I am sadder, but most times, I am both.

Although I was groggy, I could feel the stiff hospital sheets beneath my back. My hair, tucked into a blue cap, felt matted to my head. There was intense pressure. No pain. I closed my eyes and swallowed hard. My throat was dry. The nurses began to scurry, saying things like "He's perfect" and "What a beautiful boy!"

"Let me see him!" I requested urgently. The doctor lifted him up, high above the sheet that shielded me from my lower half. The baby flopped over the sheet. He was silent. He was blue.

I woke with a start in my own bed. I had somehow fallen asleep while counting kicks. Covered in sweat, I grabbed the glass of water on my nightstand and drank it quickly, trying to push the images from my mind. This dream was recurring— haunting; it replayed like an old film reel every time I nodded off, which wasn't often. As the days leading up to my scheduled C-section crept by, I wasn't able to get any real sleep. I was up counting kicks all night long, feeling for movement, poking at my belly if there was stillness for more than a minute. I thought if I went to sleep, when I woke up, my baby would be dead. I'd convinced myself that its safety was dependent on my vigilance, so I stayed perpetually tuned in, never letting my thoughts stray.

I was out of my mind with fear and I couldn't get a handle on myself. This was new for me. I was now existing in a state of constant, choking panic.

Brady and I were still sleeping in separate rooms. We were healing, but it was a slow process. There would be no picking up where we left off; we'd simply forge a new path as we moved forward to new places. I've always had a hard time holding on to anger; it was easy to forgive him but difficult to absolve myself of any wrongdoing.

Logically, I knew that his choices had nothing to do with me. They stemmed from a sad and broken place that he'd let get out of control. They weren't representative of the person he was but rather who he could become if he lost himself to that place. But there was a persistent little voice that poked at me in my worst moments, a voice that echoed all of my most hidden fears: that it really was my fault. If I had been thinner or prettier or had actually managed to get myself out of bed, put on makeup, and dress in clothes that fit; if I hadn't been so sad all of the time and hadn't depended on him to meet so many of my emotional needs, maybe he wouldn't have done it. Maybe he didn't really love me; maybe he didn't even like me. Maybe he just felt sorry for me because I had gone through some really hard shit. Maybe he didn't want to be the jerk who left the girl who'd just had her baby die but he really did want to be that guy because it meant getting away from me.

I had days when I would spiral. I would entertain all of those nasty thoughts that were truly baseless and unfounded because it was easy to feel bad, and honestly I didn't remember what it felt like to be happy anyway.

I didn't sleep for the two nights before my C-section, and my blood pressure was so high when I arrived at the hospital, my doctor said, "If we weren't having a baby today, we'd be having a baby today." But I didn't feel relief. I knew that relief wouldn't come until after the baby was out of my body and safely tucked in my arms.

Once prepped, I was wheeled into the operating room with Brady in tow. I looked over at him, dressed in a surgical gown, a cap on his head, and covers on his shoes. The protective gear they gave him had become like the uniform he wore by my side when I experienced the highest highs and the lowest lows of my life.

The anesthesiologist sat near my head, pressing buttons, allowing medicine to flow into the spinal block they'd put in, and gently uttering reassurances. I was completely numb below the waist. The room wasn't filled with music or the normal joking banter between doctors and nurses; it didn't feel jovial. It felt like they were all holding their breath. Or maybe that's just the way I felt—like I'd been underwater and holding my breath for the past year.

I felt the intense pressure as they began the procedure. My body moved slightly with each of the doctor's actions. My heart raced, my eyes teared, and I kept holding my breath.

The anesthesiologist whispered, "It's all right, don't forget to breathe." He inhaled deeply and encouraged me to breathe with him. I tried not to think about where I was or what was happening. My mind kept presenting images from the last time I'd been on my back on an operating-room table. I wondered if I would ever feel normal again or if I would forever be pulled back to that moment, over and over, to confront the trauma that my body didn't understand where to put or how to hold.

There was a lightening as they pulled the baby from my body. It was a boy.

Noah.

Brady and I had never even discussed it; we knew that, girl or boy, the name would be Noah, which means "comfort and rest." It also seemed meaningful because he was my rainbow after the storm, a promise and reminder that good things still existed.

The doctor held him up so that I could touch him, but I immediately became aware of the silence in the room. It was incredibly loud.

I heard shuffling as they rushed him over to the warmer. I ordered Brady to leave my side and go to the warmer. I could barely see the top of Noah's head, and no one would tell me what was happening.

My voice shook as I asked Brady, "What's going on?"

There was no answer.

So I spoke again, louder. "What's going on?"

"He's okay," Brady called back.

"Please, what's happening?" I asked.

"It's okay," Brady responded reassuringly.

The silence poured over me like wet cement.

Watching my blood pressure spike, the anesthesiologist whispered, "You have to calm down, you need to breathe." He ran his fingers over my forehead, scratching softly at my hairline, repeating, "Just breathe. I can see him from here. He's okay, they're just suctioning him. He probably took a little breath as he was coming out. He really is okay, I promise."

"I'm sorry," I whispered as tears leaked out of my eyes. "We lost our last baby last year. I'm really scared."

He brought his face close to mine, removed my hair covering so he could better run his fingers through my hair, and said, "I know. This time is different."

I swear that man wasn't an anesthesiologist—he was an angel.

And it *was* different.

Finally, I heard a sharp cry.

My entire body relaxed as Brady brought Noah over to me, wrapped in a blanket, and placed him in my arms. I found out later that Noah's first moments of silence were because he'd swallowed meconium during the birth. Only after the nurses cleared and suctioned his airway was he able to cry out.

As the doctor stitched me closed, I stared into Noah's eyes. There, beneath the blinding lights of the operating room, a blood pressure cuff around my upper arm, IVs in my veins, and my lower half numb, I finally came up for air.

25

Purpose

Dear Body,

Changing your habits and patterns of behavior is never easy; it's especially difficult when you do not value the thing you're changing for. In this case, body, that was you. I knew that eating well was imperative for me to lead the life I desired, but overcoming twenty-seven years of behavior was not easily accomplished. As a matter of fact, it's something I still have to work at. What makes it easier now is that I recognize and believe that I am important and so worthy, enabling me to prioritize my mental and physical health over my conditioned responses.

The relief of having Noah safely in my arms was profound.

But during the final month of my pregnancy with him, Avey, who was just four years old, was diagnosed with juvenile idiopathic arthritis. The doctors said she had been battling this condition, undiagnosed, for years. When she was just a few months old, her pediatrician and I noticed a change in her joints, but I just explained it away as being her chubby baby joints or a bumped knee or a jammed finger or growing pains.

At the beginning of 2016, right before Noah was born, we awoke to Avey screaming in pain, with every single joint in her body swollen and inflamed. Her knees looked like softballs, her finger joints like gumballs. After two days in the children's hospital and a barrage of tests, Avey finally had a diagnosis: juvenile polyarticular rheumatoid arthritis. Her inflammation markers were through the roof, and she had an erythrocyte sedimentation rate of 91, the highest the doctor had ever seen. They wanted to put her on methotrexate, a low-dose chemotherapy drug, and do steroid injections in the most affected joints. Because of her age and size, the amount and types of medication she could take were limited. We had an extremely difficult time getting her pain under control during that first month.

My sole desire was to make her well, so I began researching this autoimmune disease, inspired to figure out what could be triggering her flares and her immune system's attack on itself. My dad and Aunt Kim suffered from rheumatoid arthritis, and I knew that even when patients were medicated, they could have flare-ups that led to days, or even months, of debilitating, joint-eroding inflammation and pain.

I was highly motivated to find a way to get her off the prescribed medication and steroids and find a more holistic approach. I poured all of my being into healing Avey.

My dad was diagnosed with RA in his thirties, and he found that the weather in Texas was one of his biggest triggers. A couple of years before Avey's diagnosis, my parents moved back to California, much to my dad's relief. So when Avey began having flare-ups in the spring of 2016, we decided to experiment and see how she did in California. We were curious to see if there would be an improvement in Avey's pain levels or amount of inflammation. When Noah was only two months old, Brady shuffled me and the kids onto an airplane, and we said goodbye to him and to Texas for two weeks.

The difference in her inflammation was nearly immediate, and at the end of our two-week visit, it could not be denied. She was responding positively to the low levels of humidity and lack of barometric pressure changes; her inflammation was not just down, it was gone. Brady flew out to observe the change for himself and we knew it was time for us to make the easiest, and most difficult, decision we'd ever made.

We had to leave the life we'd built in Texas.

Brady flew back to Texas to list our grow-old-together dream house. I stayed behind in California with our three-month-old, three-year-old, and four-year-old, knowing that it was the best thing for Avey but quite possibly the worst thing for me. After years of building my own home and family, I was back where I'd started: under my parents' roof.

I was the first of my parents' seven children to get married, and as the firstborn, I'd often felt like the "trial-run" child. Having one of their children set clear boundaries with them was something my parents had never experienced before. I was met with a lot of pushback. In their eyes, if I didn't do something exactly their way, I was saying their way was wrong. But in reality, there aren't many wrong ways and there are lots of right ones. I knew that it was okay to be different, but that doesn't mean they understood it.

The friction was present on a near-daily basis. The kids and I were given the tiniest room in the house. There was barely enough space for a queen bed and a small shallow dresser. That meant I had to sleep in that bed with all three kids with our suitcases piled around the edges of it, boxes of diapers stacked on top of them. The closet was full of my mom's things and the tons of little glass knickknacks I'd res-cued from low shelves around the house before my toddlers could get their hands on them.

I didn't have money to buy the kids toys, and all my mom had was mega-blocks, books, and a baby bouncer. I tried to find ways to entertain them without resorting to various screens, but my parents' house was the same way it had al-ways been: The TV was constantly on and blaring. If I made a comment or asked if I could turn it off, I was met with eye-rolling and refusal.

Avey was on a special diet. After she was diagnosed, I de-cided to put our entire family on the autoimmune protocol diet, a highly restrictive diet that minimizes inflammatory foods like grains, dairy, legumes, nightshades, nuts, seeds, eggs, and anything with refined or processed ingredients. Since giv-ing birth to Noah and starting this diet, I had lost sixty-eight pounds, so my mom was excited about it—she said that we'd all go on the "Avey diet"—and I agreed to cook for my par-ents as well. But they only lasted about a week; after that, they began to order in, even if I'd already prepared food. Mealtime became a constant source of tension. The kids wanted to eat what their uncles—I still had three younger brothers living at home—and grandparents were eating, but we had seen some success on this diet for Avey, and I didn't want to lose momen-tum or backslide.

I was struggling to take care of myself, and things grew tense between my mom and me. She would disapprove of something I did or said, and instead of changing my behavior as I had in the past, I held my ground, which she wasn't used to—and didn't like—and which caused her to lose her tem-per. If I asked her to lower her voice, she would tell me not to tell her what to do in her own house. So my only choice was to shuffle the children outside because they weren't used to that type of behavior, and it scared and confused them.

The mom who'd cared for me so lovingly when Elias passed away was lost in grief over him too. She was the person who'd taught me to turn to food for comfort, and I was watching her deal with loss by doing the same thing.

Of course, being around that every day, I saw all the work I'd done to regain a healthy relationship with food go out the window. Under pressure and back in my most triggering place, I returned to self-sabotaging behavior. And I was slowly breaking under the weight of caring for three children around the clock with no one to turn to for help. Noah had really bad acid reflux, so I was constantly shuffling everyone to doctors' appointments, and I felt like I never got a break. I felt trapped, isolated, and very alone. I had never gone through a postpartum period without a partner who was wholly present and willing to help in whatever ways he could. I was still desperately sad about losing Elias, and although Noah brought comfort, he wasn't a replacement. I was still learning how to navigate the world with this huge gaping hole in the center of me.

How did people do this?

How did they keep going on?

It all felt so impossible and meaningless.

I could feel myself slipping away every day, my anxiety and depression colliding in a vortex of sorrow. My already fragile mental state began to decline further; after Elias died, I'd sometimes thought that I wished I had died with him, and lately began to wish I could die now.

One night as I lay in bed with all of the kids surrounding me, the TV blaring down the hall in the living room, and my youngest brother's music blasting from the room above me,

I began to plan it all out. I'd leave the kids with my mom, tell her I was going to a doctor's appointment, and then I'd drive. I'd drive on I-5 along the coast, with all of its treacherous mountain roads. I'd meander for a bit, taking in the sight of the ocean and the smell of the surf, and then I'd just coast right off the side. It would look like an accident, so no one would have to live with the fact that I had made this choice. People wouldn't have to wonder whether it was their fault that I was no longer living—they'd only have to deal with the loss. I was convinced everyone would be better off without me. Even though Brady and I were much stronger at that point, I told myself that he'd be happier with another wife—someone more attractive, better at housework, better at making him happy. The state I was in reminded me of how I'd been in the weeks leading up to Noah's birth. I was spinning and spinning and couldn't rein myself in.

While I watched the ceiling fan turn and fantasized about how I'd kill myself, my phone, beside me on the bed, began to buzz softly. It was Brady. I felt caught, knowing that if I answered, I'd tell him how I was feeling. And I knew if I told him, I wouldn't ever be able to act on my plan. I answered before I had much time to think about it.

"Hey, babe," he said. "I'm headed to bed, just wanted to call to say good night."

I took a breath and whispered, "I need to tell you something."

And then I unburdened myself. I told him all the ways I was struggling. I knew that Brady was shocked and deeply concerned. He told me the truth: that I was loved and that he couldn't imagine not having me in his life; that no one could ever love our kids or raise them as well as I could; that it was okay to feel sad and maybe what I really needed was to learn how to get comfortable sitting with sadness instead of always trying to escape it; and that I had a purpose, that there was purpose to all of it—everything I'd gone through—and maybe that purpose was of greater design, maybe I was supposed to help other people.

As I listened to him, I realized that I'd been entertaining lies. I'd become so disappointed in my body and my circumstances that I'd paved a path in my mind that led to hate. *Come right in, loathing. Have a seat, anger. Can I offer you any tea?* You can't heal a body you hate, but you can poison it, and that's exactly what I'd done. It had become easy to believe the lies because they were the thoughts I dwelled on and rehearsed.

While I know there are thousands of platforms that help people manage the treacherous roads of depression, grief, and trauma, we didn't have any money for a psychiatrist, and I didn't have time to read a book, so instead, I chose to confide in those people around me who felt like healers and who would continue to point me toward the truth. After that conversation with Brady, I never thought about ending my life again. That thought was banished to the depths, where it belonged. But something he said that night stuck with me. When he told me I had a purpose, something sparked within me, something I had forgotten, something I knew I needed to keep at the surface so I could figure out what it was and give it to the world.

26

Change

Dear Body,
    You have always tried to communicate with me, but it was in a language I did not understand until later in life. I'm sorry it took me so long to figure out how to listen.

And I said to my body. Softly. "I want to be your friend."
—NAYYIRAH WAHEED, "THREE"

On October 31, 2016, Brady finally made his way out to California, and our family was whole once again. Initially, we moved into corporate housing, a little high-rise apartment in La Jolla. It was one of the smallest places we'd ever lived, but we embraced the positive things about it, like living within walking distance of an amazing outdoor mall, having only a twenty-minute drive to the ocean, and being surrounded by restaurants that delivered (this was before the days of Door-Dash and Uber Eats).

We were allowed to live in the apartment for sixty days while we looked for a house. I found a lot of joy within those walls. Even though it was a small two-bedroom on the fourth floor, it was more space and freedom than I'd had in the past six months. It felt nice to be together again, not to have to worry about taking up someone else's space or being a burden. I felt lighter just being out of my parents' house. Even though the situation was temporary, it represented the future.

For the first time in a decade, I spent Thanksgiving in California. My sister flew in from Texas, and everyone was grateful to be celebrating the holiday together in such beautiful weather. After dinner, my sister called me into my mom's small downstairs guest bathroom.

"I'm going to do your makeup," she exclaimed as she bounced excitedly, mascara and foundation gripped tightly in her hands. "Don't say no!" she quickly added.

I took in the sight of my baby sister, no longer a baby at twenty-two. She was tall and slender, wearing a spectacular dress, and made up beautifully, like a Kardashian or a model. I was always so impressed with her makeup expertise. I remembered back when I was a teenager, I used to feel so excited about getting ready for school. I planned and coordinated everything perfectly, down to the color eyeshadow that I would wear each day.

I used to get compliments on my hair all the time, but it had been years since I'd bothered getting it cut or styling it. Brady had been cutting my hair, if you can believe that! But back in my teens and early twenties, before the invention of Pinterest, I would save photos from the internet in a file on my desktop and write meticulously detailed notes in a journal after observing styles from movies or shows I especially liked. I used to be so passionate about all of it—it brought me so much joy. But somewhere along the way, I had lost that joy. It stopped mattering. *I* stopped mattering. You don't invest time and energy into things that you don't care about.

I sat down with a smile and extended my arms. "Make me pretty," I requested.

"Oh, you have the pretty part down," she said as she began to mix foundation colors to match my skin tone. "This is just to make you glow."

It was an hour I'll never forget—me trying to sneak peeks at the mirror and her reprimanding me, the two of us talking about boys and life and how hard things can be. We paused from time to time to shout song lyrics at the tops of our lungs and dance silly. And during that hour, something began to come back to life inside me, something I hadn't felt since becoming a wife and a mother, something I'd thought I'd lost as I got older. Now I realized that maybe it wasn't lost; it was just buried under all the other things that I thought mattered more. In that moment, I truly couldn't recall why I'd stopped thinking that nurturing this part of myself was important.

"You have such beautiful eyes," she remarked as she applied mascara in perfect strokes to my eyelashes.

"They're the same color as yours," I murmured.

"Like I said, beautiful," she whispered. "Okay," she said louder. She stood up and clapped her hands. "That's it! You're finished, and I am brilliant!" She stepped back to admire her work. "You look incredible!"

I turned to face the mirror, and I felt like I was seeing someone whom I had loved very much at one time, long ago. The years melted away, and I was reminded that I still loved her so greatly; it was as if I had forgotten her and was now seeing her again for the first time in a long while.

Her. Oh, I do remember her.
That girl who could do anything, be anything.

My sister was right—she had made me glow. She'd relit a fire within me that I hadn't known had gone out, and it was something I didn't want to lose sight of or let go of ever again. After that evening, I began to set time aside for myself to invest in the little things that made me feel good. It started with a trip that very night to Ulta to begin to rebuild a makeup stash because all I had at that point was three-dollar CoverGirl powder, eyeliner, mascara, and ChapStick.

In the weeks and months that followed, the first thing I did when I got up was put on a little shimmer. Getting dressed and putting on makeup in the morning—taking ten to fifteen minutes to do something nice for myself—changed the tone of my whole day. I was suddenly more productive than I'd been in years. I was motivated to accomplish tasks and even get out of the house more. I bought clothes that fit me at the size I was instead of waiting to lose weight. That alone completely changed the way I felt in my body. Sure, the clothes were size 22 and XXL, but the size hardly mattered to me anymore. They weren't tight or restricting. I'd forgotten how good it felt to wear clothes that fit!

I began to regain my self-esteem. By doing small things for my body and mental well-being, showing myself that I cared, I was actually starting to believe that I was someone important enough to do those things for. I respected and responded to my most basic needs, and it felt so good that I started actively listening to my body, my heart, and my soul to try to find more ways I could nurture myself. I took pride in who I was becoming. It is so easy to define your identity as someone who takes care of everyone else, but you can't pour from an empty cup. In disregarding my own well-being, I was diminishing my capacity to care for others. When I took a little time for myself, the quality of my time spent caring for others increased in value.

I cannot stress enough how important the little things are. I hadn't lost a hundred pounds. I hadn't made drastic changes to my diet or increased my level of activity. I was simply accepting myself exactly where I was and embracing the life that I found myself in, even though it looked different from how I had imagined it would. I was choosing to bloom where I had been planted instead of constantly fighting it.

And so I bloomed.

After a few months of searching, in December 2016, we found a house just outside San Diego. It was a new build on two and a half acres of land, which was more important to us than the house itself.

We moved in right before Christmas. I was excited to have my own kitchen again, restock our pantry, get away from all the takeout food we'd been eating for nearly a year. I hadn't wanted to begin another diet change and invest in stocking our kitchen until our living situation was more stable. As a result, in the past year, my weight had dropped from 260 pounds down to 188 pounds and then bounced back up to over 220.

I was excited for the new year and a fresh start. As I ate better, I began to feel better physically and mentally. I think that being reunited with Brady and resuming raising our kids together instead of single-moming it was a huge part of it too. I knew I had to learn more about health and wellness. I wanted to learn how to create recipes for my family that suited our dietary needs. I also wanted recipes that didn't require us to triple our grocery budget and change our palates entirely.

I've found that when you're on a weight-loss journey, many

resources tell you to cut out some of the most affordable foods in the grocery store, like rice, beans, potatoes, and even fruit! That felt like impractical advice that lacked long-term sense. I figured that if I was going to make a sustainable lifestyle change, cutting out everything that made food enjoyable or affordable—including dressings and sauces that go along with it—would set me up for failure. I knew that, armed with the right equipment, I could become successful at re-creating all the foods we loved by using simple ingredient swaps that increased nutritional value.

While I was expanding my general understanding of food and how it affected my family's life, there were still everyday things that needed to be figured out. The first was how to cook more meals at home. Though not having time to cook was an excuse I'd made for years, cooking at home really did involve a fair amount of time and planning. Like everyone else, I take pride in creating a meal for the people I love, but it's still a chore that requires effort.

A couple of years earlier, I'd decided to take my cooking skills to the next level. After reading about the harmful toxins found in the lining of cans, such as BPA, and the high amounts of sodium in canned food—not to mention the toll all those cans were taking on our landfills—I started making our own canned beans at home. My friend AlinaJoy was able to reduce her family of five's grocery budget to just five hundred dollars a month by getting rid of convenience foods and canning things at home. One day she showed me her handy-dandy stove-top pressure cooker that she used to cook dry beans, and I was hooked!

I immediately went home and spoke with Brady about buying one. I was pregnant with Elias at the time and I asked him if he wouldn't mind doing the research for me on the best one to buy. He readily agreed. Not long after, he proudly sat me in front of his computer and showed me the tool he swore would make all my bean dreams come true. It was an Instant Pot, a spaceship-like thing that had so many buttons and knobs, it looked ridiculous. At the time, the gadget was relatively unknown, with only about thirty reviews on Amazon. As Brady showed it to me, he talked excitedly about all the features it had.

"It's not just a pressure cooker! It's a yogurt maker, a steamer, a rice cooker. You can sauté right in the pot to reduce your dishes—it does so much!"

"Yes, it does," I said, trying to keep my tone even, "but it costs one million dollars and I don't need any of those functions. I'm not making yogurt; I just want to make beans. Can we please just go with the simple stove-top option?" I was exaggerating, of course; back then, the Instant Pot was $120, but it might as well have been a million to me.

Brady responded, "I promise this one is better, you'll see!"

Three days later, Brady came into the house, strutting like a peacock, with a multicolored box in hand.

"You didn't."

"I did." He smiled.

"Baaaabe," I moaned. "I just wanted a simple little pressure cooker; I don't want to have to learn another thing!" I was pregnant and miserable, experiencing severe breastfeeding aversion. Benjamin was still nursing around the clock, and it felt like nails on a chalkboard, if that was a feeling you could have in your nipples. I didn't want to learn the alien language of a fancy new gadget. I just wanted to cook some beans. But now I was the proud owner of a countertop appliance that looked like it was made by NASA. He set it on the floor of the living room. I gave it the side-eye. *He'll see, buying that pot was a mistake. He'll see.*

A couple of weeks later, the pot still stared at me from

its position next to the lime-green hand-me-down recliner. Brady came into the room, buttoning his shirt for work, as I nursed Ben while gritting my teeth.

He sighed. "So you're not even gonna try it, eh?"

"It was a hundred and twenty dollars, Brady." I paused for dramatic effect. "Before tax."

He chuckled. "But if it lasts us ten years, isn't it worth it?"

I frowned.

"Okay, okay. If you don't use it by the end of the day, I'll return it," he said. He kissed us all and left for work.

That pot and I were in a standoff until lunchtime, when I started to experience an odd feeling that felt a little bit like remorse. Was I being ungrateful? *Could* this be the better option? I rolled my eyes, grabbed the box, and cut through the tape.

I'll just read the manual, I decided. *See what it's all about.* Suddenly, operating the machine didn't seem so hard. I washed the pot and decided to make rice first. After all, if I ruined a little bit of rice, what was the harm?

My toddlers licked their bowls and asked for more! Even I enjoyed my portion and I sent Brady a picture, admitting defeat.

My romance with the Instant Pot started slowly. But before I knew it, I was navigating the functions like a pro. I was browning proteins, adding other ingredients, and expertly setting the cook time after snapping the lid in place. Soups, casseroles, salad toppers, spaghetti, lasagna—you name it, I could make it, and in a fraction of the time it took in an oven or on a stove top!

And the fact that it was so hands-off was the best part. I would throw half a dozen vegetables in the pot, pop the top in place, push two buttons, walk away, and in thirty minutes, I'd come back and have a healthy dinner waiting to be served.

I didn't have to worry about the stove being on or water boiling in pots within arm's reach of little ones. Everything was contained, sealed shut. Even the space it took up wasn't an issue. Once I'd popped all the ingredients into the pot, I'd push it into a corner and get all my counter space back.

The Instant Pot eliminated my biggest excuse for not eating healthy: that I didn't have the time. With the pot doing all the work for me, I could go do laundry, change diapers, breastfeed, burp babies, or tackle housework. When the food was done cooking, we could have dinner then or I could leave it on the Keep Warm setting until we were ready to eat. That meant I was able to make dinner at two in the afternoon, which was my magical time. The kids were getting up from their naps and I'd let them watch a show; I'd put Benjamin in the baby carrier on my back and quickly chop up some things, throw them in the pot, then set it back. Once it was done, I'd leave it on Keep Warm until Brady got home from work at five thirty and we'd all have dinner together. This silly gadget that I'd once envisioned throwing off the top of a mountain was changing my life in more positive ways than I could count.

In December 2016, as I stood barefoot in the middle of my new kitchen, I grinned as I ripped the packing tape off the brown moving box labeled INSTANT POT. Reverently, like pulling a diamond out of the earth, I unpacked my electric pressure cooker. I blew the dust off the lid, carefully wiped the sides with a washcloth, and set it proudly on the quartz countertop.

Oh yeah, change was a-coming.

27

Power to Heal

Dear Body,
  I've always been in awe of your incredible ability
to heal—little cuts and scrapes, blemishes, and
broken bones. The power of healing you hold is
immense and impressive; I just never realized quite
how much until I began giving you the tools required
to heal big things, like autoimmune disease, chronic
inflammation, skin rashes, insomnia, and bowel
disorders. You are truly a wonder.

At the beginning of 2017, just a couple weeks after moving
into our new home, I was craving a positive challenge to usher
in the new year. Instead of declaring yet another weight-loss
resolution (because, let's be honest, they had not worked so
well in the past), I decided to take my focus off my weight and
place it on my habits. I challenged myself to cook a whole-
foods dinner at home every night for an entire year. With
my time excuse eliminated, a new kitchen and environment to

cook in, and all the knowledge I'd acquired over the years, I knew I could get us eating more at home and less out of a box. With the Instant Pot, our other kitchen gadgets, and my hardened determination, I was going to accomplish my goal.

I started trying to create sweet and savory recipes that suited our preferences, working around our kids' food allergies and aversions. There were a couple of things we had to steer clear of for Avey. I limited our dairy intake but didn't cut it out entirely. I began viewing dairy in a different light—as a condiment instead of a mainstay. Dairy can cause inflammation in the body, and autoimmune diseases are inflammatory diseases. It seemed clear that our bodies handle it better in small doses, so we tried consuming less. I liked cheese on my salad and sprinkled on roasted broccoli as a snack. We even continued to eat enchiladas, lasagna, and pizza; I just sprinkled lightly!

We agreed to get rid of artificial sugars, and if there was an ingredient on the nutritional label that we couldn't pronounce or understand clearly, we opted for something else. One of the ways I transitioned my family to this kind of eating was by involving them. I figured if this was important enough for me to learn to give them the best quality of health and life, then it was something I should be teaching them as well. In teaching them, I was encouraged to learn more and deepen my understanding of nutrition and what ingredients were actually in the foods we ate. Because of this, my kids have been reading labels since they were five and six years old.

We sat our kids down and explained that we had not always made the best or most appropriate food choices, that food mattered, and that when God created the world, He gave us all the food we needed in order to thrive. Our bodies change on a cellular level based on what we eat. Our diets can even influence what genes are expressed through epigenetics, or the way DNA is influenced by lifestyle factors. In other words, we literally are what we eat. McDonald's certainly tastes good, but fast-food chicken nuggets and French fries don't build healthy, well-nourished bodies. We asked them to give us grace as we all learned how to navigate this new territory together.

We didn't throw out all of our food; we simply consumed what we had, and when it was gone, we replaced it with better choices. There are people who will tell you that if you're using a salad dressing that contains high-fructose syrup, it negates the benefit of the salad. It doesn't. You can use a salad dressing that doesn't have the best ingredients in it and still succeed at weight loss. You're still getting the benefits of all those delicious fibrous vegetables. But as you grow in your nutrition knowledge, something I'm still doing, you begin to do better. You replace the old with the new. This is not an all-or-nothing thing, nor does it happen overnight. Wellness is cumulative; it builds on itself. So maybe on day one of your health journey, you use Hidden Valley Ranch, but then on day forty-two, when you hit the end of the bottle, you replace it with a homemade or store-bought version that's nutritionally better for you. One thing doesn't necessarily negate the other. It's not black or white. I choose not to sweat the small stuff. I did the best I could when I could and strove to learn more as I went along.

All of the choices we make for our well-being add up, whether it's a season where we're focusing on our mental health and growth, a season where we're focusing on specific food ingredients, water intake, and sleep, or a season where we really dig deep to find the energy to move more. One builds on the other. Sometimes it's better to do one thing well than a lot of things just so-so. I've learned it's best to narrow your focus and start with one thing.

Start with food.

I chose to begin to value myself in the same way I'd been valuing and loving my children for years. Just because a toddler wants to eat three ice cream cones in one sitting doesn't mean he should or that I should let him. No, the poor guy is going to get all hopped up on sugar, act like a fool, and be left with a bellyache. As parents who know it's not a wise thing to do, we have to save them from their own lack of wisdom.

In the same way, just because I want to eat an entire value-size bag of Doritos doesn't mean that's wise for me. The MSG alone would probably leave me with an awful headache; the corn would make me gassy; and my stomach wouldn't feel too happy about having to digest an entire pound of fake nacho flavoring. It's easy to tell our children no. It's much more difficult to tell ourselves no and exercise that same kind of discipline over our own choices—especially when dealing with food and emotional triggers. This is why I also decided it was time to do the emotional work too. Admittedly, I'm still working on it.

I didn't have a weight problem. I had a self-medicating problem. I had a self-worth and a self-respect problem. I had learned behaviors and responses that I needed to heal, past trauma to overcome. I was dealing with subconscious coping mechanisms that had been carefully crafted over years and years. I had an unhealthy relationship with food, and I know I'm not alone in that. Most people who lose weight regain it within a year. It is said that 95 percent of people who lose weight regain it all within five years. It's not as simple as energy consumed and expended. I didn't have a weight problem, and the sooner I acknowledged, understood, and accepted that, the sooner I could cut through the crud and begin to heal.

Around this time, I finally grasped that food was the key to so much more than health. Through nurturing our bodies and eating whole, unprocessed foods, our family felt better overall. We had lower levels of toxins in our systems. We had less inflammation because we ate fewer preservatives. There also came a sense of pride in doing something that felt so natural, practicing an art form that had existed from the beginning of humankind.

I had come to a place where I understood just how intuitive the body was. I figured if I could embrace the concept that food is love and insist on nourishing my body with that love, my body would respond in kind. Looking back, I see that self-compassion really was the key to my success. When you're dieting, people think you have to be in a militant mindset all the time. That kind of thinking can really set you up for disaster. No one can be *on* all the time, and the ramifications of internal criticism often wreak havoc on the body; the stress can actually increase inflammation.

One of the ways I simplified this new way of eating was by establishing a degree of familiarity with the foods we bought. If you know anything about what I do, you might think what I'm about to tell you is crazy, but I don't love meal planning. In fact, I'd go so far as to say it sucks the life out of me. I found a middle ground by creating a familiar route in the grocery store, buying the same list of nutrient-packed foods over and over, and adding a new fruit or veggie to the mix every other week. Instead of using those foods the same way every time, I found new ways to incorporate them into dishes we'd never eaten before.

As our year of exclusively eating at home progressed, weight began coming off me like it never had before. I couldn't believe the difference it was making in all areas of my life. Once I'd figured out recipes my family and I loved and learned how to fully utilize the Instant Pot, it took very little effort to make delicious, filling meals that were also packed with nutrients.

In my excitement, I decided to post something in my Crunchy Breastfeeders group on Facebook, a holistic mothers' group that I co-administrated while I was in Texas. Even though we had moved across the country, I still considered those women to be my community. Someone asked about losing weight while breastfeeding. I explained how I'd been eating whole foods and decreasing portion sizes. In the post, I mentioned that I'd lost forty-six pounds in three months, was feeling great, and that my milk supply was unaffected.

Immediately, women in the group started asking me questions, so I excitedly told them about the Instant Pot. I explained what a cool gadget it was and how it looked intimidating but was really the most magical thing ever. My fingers flew as I typed, telling them all the ways it had improved my life.

Someone in the group mentioned that I should share my story on the Instant Pot Facebook page and that people in the group would love it. So I checked the page out. At that time, the community was small, with only two hundred thousand people in the group (compared to the millions it has today). As I scrolled, I noticed that there was no one in the group posting about healthy foods. It seemed everyone was making ribs, mac and cheese, or cheesecake in their pots. I posted side-by-side before-and-after pictures of myself and a story about what I was doing. I told them how I was just a mom who loved my Instant Pot and that I wanted to encourage people to try tackling healthier recipes in the pot because the benefits were amazing.

Immediately, the post went viral. I couldn't even get my Facebook to open because I had so many notifications pouring in. I started responding to thousands and thousands of comments on the post. Then I began receiving personal messages. People wanted to know:

How are you doing it?
What are your recipes?
How can I have the same success?
Do you have a cookbook?

Brady was out of town on business, so I called him and said, "I'm not sure, but I think something is happening."

As we talked, I noticed that I suddenly had thousands of friend requests. Within moments, I received a notification from Facebook that they were going to shut my page down because they thought I was doing something illegal due to all the action on my page over such a short period. I quickly posted in the thread that people should stop friending and messaging me for just a little bit while I figured out an alternative. I realized that I needed to do something. But what should that be? Was I ready?

28

Crossroads

Dear Body,

When we work in tandem, we have the ability to accomplish great things! I wasted so much time fighting you instead of coming alongside you to support your needs and love you right where you were. The way I want to be loved by others is the same way you want to be loved by me.

At this moment, I could sense I was at a crossroads. I had this feeling that something big was on the horizon, but it was too far off to spot just yet. I couldn't help but wonder if I was beginning to see it come into focus. Though at that point, I never could have guessed what it would turn into. All I knew was that if I could help one person though a rough spot, then maybe everything I'd gone through, all the ups and the downs, the peaks and the valleys, had a purpose.

I didn't give it a second thought; I created a Facebook community to share everything I'd learned and why I was finally having lasting success in my very long journey to health.

I sat and thought for a moment and decided to put *Instant Pot* and *weight loss* together and called it the Instant Loss community. Within the first couple of hours, more than two thousand people joined the group, and it just kept growing and growing and growing and growing. I crafted this message that I pinned to the top of the page:

Hi, and welcome to the Instant Loss community. I'm so glad you're here! I'm Brittany and I'm happy to share with you the intense joy I've gotten out of discovering ways to eat healthy using my Instant Pot. I have always struggled with my weight, my relationship with food, my body, and my health. I became a chronic dieter. I was desperate to try anything to feel better but I never found sustainable success until now. When quick-fix pills, shakes, premade meals, and diets failed, there was always an excuse, always a reason to put my health on the back burner. I often thought to myself that my weight was my biggest problem in life, but I've finally realized that weight was never really my problem at all . . . it was merely a symptom of a much deeper issue. The process of getting to the root of a lot of those problems and working through those things was happening in tandem with my shift into eating better. I began to maintain a whole foods diet as I taught myself about nutrition. When someone asks what my diet is, I simply reply, "J.E.R.F." It means "Just eat real food." Simple but incredibly effective. I've done so much healing in the past few months, and as funny as it sounds, my Instant Pot is at the center of it all.

The message seemed to resonate with a lot of people; it got them excited and offered hope. I started posting recipes in the Facebook group. Very quickly, though, within the first twenty-four hours, people started voicing their displeasure with this method. One message read, "This is not going to work. You need to have a blog. Because everyone is commenting and introducing themselves, your recipes keep getting pushed to the bottom of the feed."

A blog? A website? These things seemed completely out of reach at the time, impossible to achieve. *How?* I needed to call in the troops.

I called my friend AlinaJoy. She was the only successful blogger who I knew at the time. She talked to me for two hours, encouraging me, telling me that I could learn how to do it, that it wasn't really that hard. While I was on the phone with her, she said, "You're going to buy the domain while you are on the phone with me. I'm making sure that you do this."

The second I clicked Buy, a wave of nerves swept over me. I knew I'd need to spend a hundred and fifty dollars for all the necessities to start the blog. One hundred and fifty dollars seemed like a lot to gamble on a Facebook comment. Our two-week grocery budget was one hundred and fifty dollars.

That night, I watched YouTube videos on how to make a blog and began piecing it all together. I stayed up two nights in a row building the website. Noah was still nursing through the night at that point, and Avey and Ben were both under five. Through nursing, calming crying kiddos, and lulling little ones back to sleep after nightmares, I built Instant Loss's very first website. I don't even remember how—I just tried to be a sponge, soaking up as much information as possible; I told the group that I had no idea what I was doing and asked for grace. I knew this wasn't going to be a smooth process. I launched the site and crossed my fingers.

To my surprise, as clunky as the site was, it worked.

Traffic was high out of the gate: fifty-two thousand hits the first day, and the growth was continuous. And as things grew, I became more and more excited about all the inspiration and information I was able to offer. Instant Loss was a round-the-clock, 24/7 job. I spent six to eight hours every day just responding to messages, e-mails, and comments. I let people into our home via livestreams as I encouraged them to cook lunch with me, make homemade pasta, and have kitchen dance parties, all with a tiny baby on my back and small children at my feet. I was posting a recipe a day on the blog, taking photos with my iPhone 5, and uploading raw images; I literally didn't have a clue. But I think people found that appealing, because it was real. It was clear I didn't have ulterior motives; I was literally the group cheerleader. I just wanted everyone to feel as great as I did.

The first weekend the website was live, we exceeded our traffic for the entire month. I had to pay another ninety dollars just to get the host to turn my server back on. I quickly realized that blogging wasn't cheap and I needed to do something to at least break even. I was working nearly eighteen hours a day, and while I was extremely inspired to continue helping others, I couldn't see how I could keep up that pace, especially for free.

One night, as I scoured the web for articles on ways bloggers can make money, I came across a really great piece. The author pointed out that the only way you'll ever make serious cash blogging is to market something that nobody else has and that people want from *you*—something no one else can give them. Keeping this in mind, I started to make a list of things everybody had asked me for. Then I thought about what on that list was something that only I could give them. It was a light-bulb moment.

Meal plans.

As I began building my first meal plan, I told Brady, "If I only make six hundred dollars off this, it will be worth my time and I'll feel compensated for the effort I've put in." I priced it at $3.99. I wanted it to be affordable for everyone. Over the years, I had seen so many plans I wanted to purchase but that were too expensive. Who has $280 for a weight-loss plan? I didn't even have that for groceries! I posted it on the blog, announced it in the Facebook group, and said a quick prayer. Then I waited.

In the first hour, I made $2,000.

In the first day, I made $4,200.

In the first month, I made $8,000.

In the first year, during which I expanded to six meal plans, I'd made over $100,000.

That sounds crazy, right?

It felt crazy to be living it!

I started creating bundle deals where people could bundle different meal plans. This way, buyers could bundle a month's worth of meal plans for an entire family, plus grocery lists, for fifteen dollars. People loved them. The best part? People actually followed them. Tons of people in the group were losing weight, just like I was. All of a sudden, I had testimony after testimony after testimony from people who were following my plans and my recipes and doing what I was doing. They were losing weight while getting free from food addiction, binge eating, and other harmful food-related behaviors.

The excitement was electric.

I was in full-out go mode, running on pure joy. I didn't sleep. I didn't take a moment to rest. I spent all my time creating Instagram stories and posts encouraging my people. They call them followers, but they had really become my friends. Because I loved them all so deeply, and I knew what it felt like to give up, I was dedicated to responding to every comment, every message. I just wanted them to know that they were seen, that even if the rest of the world wasn't listening, I was.

But responding to tens of thousands of people was a full-time job in itself. I value treating others the way I want to be treated, and I was all too familiar with those desperate dark places that many were coming to me from. I'd been there. I'd experienced it. I knew exactly what it felt like to be an island, overweight, and lost in a sea of other people's opinions. I never wanted anybody to feel like I didn't hear them, see them, know them, or empathize with them. It didn't matter that I was running a more-than-full-time business, raising my kids, cloth-diapering, making every meal from scratch, and busting my butt as a stay-at-home mom. I could do it because they needed me to do it.

News spread quickly about my platform and the success my followers were having. Four months after Instant Loss took off, the *Chicago Tribune* wrote a story about me. Then, to my surprise, the *New York Times* picked it up. After that, it snowballed. The *LA Times* reported on it, then *Good Morning America* called.

That's when Instant Loss went national.

Good Morning America asked me to do an interview in my home—a segment all about the Instant Pot. They made it seem like it was going to be all about me, my story, and Instant Loss, but really, it was just a commercial for the Instant Pot—the hottest Black Friday item of the year! It didn't matter in the end, though, because that TV appearance catapulted Instant Loss from a homemade website into something much bigger.

29

Life of Nevers

Dear Body,
  We have big dreams and aspirations, but we cannot be all things to all people. Part of taking care of ourselves means respecting the fact that we are only human and allowing ourselves to be authentic. Rest is part of the work. Growth is part of the work. Unabashed honesty with oneself is part of the work.

Life had become a chaotic, beautiful mess. *Rachael Ray, The Doctors, People* magazine, and *Better Homes and Gardens* called. The Hallmark Channel even sent me an e-mail. All the while, I was still trying to juggle being a full-time mom, supporting more than seventy thousand people on social media, answering every private message, replying to every comment, publishing new recipes, and cheerleading those who were having success or needed an extra bit of encouragement. I was continuously reminded to take time to replenish and recharge. You can't pour from an empty cup, but filling that cup is easier said than done.

I was running at a breakneck pace, seizing this rare moment of opportunity that most people never get even if they work their whole lives for it. I knew what was happening was very special. I also realized that when the spotlight finds you, it won't be long before it moves on and finds someone else. I became a "yes man." Respond to every comment and every message? Yes! Build a business empire while simultaneously working as a stay-at-home mom? Yes! Continue to lose weight in front of now hundreds of thousands of people? Yes! The business end wasn't sucking the life out of me; it was actually kindling something inside me, something that surprised me, because it ran counter to a fundamental part of who I was and who I thought I wanted to be.

I didn't want to be a stay-at-home mom.

I wanted to be a working mom.

My mom's greatest desire from the time she was a child was to be a stay-at-home mother. Because she married at such a young age and because of her often tumultuous relationship with my dad, she had to figure out a way to care for us kids financially on her own. During the first six or so years of their marriage, my parents were on again, off again. He lived with his mom, cities away, and my mom lived with her parents while she attended nursing school. She applied to programs that could help her stay on her feet, like welfare, and got financial aid to help pay for school.

While she loved my dad, staying with him meant sacrificing the desires of her heart—to stay home with us. This caused her to feel resentment and bitterness toward my dad and the people around her who had the life she wanted for herself. Growing up, I believed that being a stay-at-home parent was the only way to prevent that bitterness from taking root within me. At sixteen, I felt like I knew everything. I thought I was capable of being a wife and a mother, but looking back through older, wiser eyes, I'm so glad I didn't end up obtaining the desires of my youth. With age comes maturity, and with maturity, a clearer vision. It's funny how kids think they know everything, but maturing is being able to admit that you really know nothing at all, and the things that you do know are subject to change; they evolve and expand past your points of certainty.

As a kid, I envisioned how awesome it would be to have a mom who was home all the time to take care of you, make you dinner, and joyfully help with homework, laughing over math problems as you shared snacks and took breaks to gossip. As an adult, I realize just how unsuited my mom was for the role I always imagined her in. She is an amazing, driven, resilient woman who provided in abundance for her family. But I don't believe she would have been nearly as satisfied staying home, doing laundry, and baking bread as she always believed she'd be.

I speak from experience. Because sometimes you get everything you ever wanted and then realize it wasn't really what you wanted at all.

In many ways, my childhood trauma has left me uncertain as a mother. I've struggled with physical intimacy and emotional vulnerability. I can get so triggered in the moment that I give my children confusing or hard-to-understand messages. I'm so afraid of inflicting trauma or creating lasting scars that sometimes, honestly, it's easier to walk away and avoid dealing with problems.

When I was nine, my dad went on medical disability and became the stay-at-home parent. He and I were like two peas in a pod; we got along really well because our personalities were so similar. Although we spent a lot of time together laughing, bonding, enjoying that father-daughter love, there was a dark side to our relationship. He was often in pain, and living with the frustration of his own circumstances spilled into tremendous overreactions when dealing with us kids and our mistakes. He'd often tell us, "Shit flows downhill," by which he meant that he got shit from my mom, so he gave us shit. I know that this should have made me angry with my dad, but it was easier to be angry with my mom—if she wasn't so mean to my dad, he wouldn't have been so mean to us. I now recognize this manipulation for what it was.

I had a difficult time relating to my mom and felt that if she was home more, things would be easier. As an adult, I realize that I was wrong. My mom and I are more similar than I sometimes like to admit. I come from a long line of working women—my great-grandma, my grandma, my mom, and now me. Though some might see this as gender-role reversal, I honestly feel like there are just some women out there who kick butt in the workforce. It simply shouldn't be taboo to have one spouse work while the other stays at home, regardless of gender.

It's acceptable, sometimes even expected, in our society for a woman to be a stay-at-home parent. But society isn't always as understanding if a man wants to take on that very same role. He may be seen as failing in his duties as a man. Even worse, people may think he's letting his family down. This is just not the truth. Human beings are complex, and we are all so very different. Not all men are built to be financial providers, just like not all women are built to be primary caregivers.

Nowadays, this is a more accepted truth. But back in the 1960s or the 1930s, it was rare for the primary breadwinner to be a woman. My mom is an amazing organizer. When there is something to be planned, accomplished, or taken care of, she is the one you call. And she is meticulous, detailed-oriented, and leaves no stone unturned. My mother is highly intelligent, an expert communicator—she can wear all the hats, but she is not a nurturer. It's not her nature.

I embraced the role of primary caregiver and I was grateful for it, but my heart longed for something else. While I deeply appreciated having the choice to stay home, it wasn't ideal for me. Internally, I warred with what was expected of me and what I knew I truly wanted.

But there was a lot of soul work I had to do before I could admit that to myself.

Brady hated the nine-to-five life—it's not in his blood. He has the credentials of an engineer but the heart of a farmer and an inventor. When I first started earning money, it was easier for me to frame it as something I was doing for *him* instead of something I was doing for myself. Earning money so that my husband didn't have to was just another way of being a supportive wife, of helping to create the life of his dreams.

I hid behind that idea instead of owning the fact that I really love to work and would rather do that than be a homemaker. I simply couldn't say that out loud. It felt like a betrayal of who I *should* be and what I *should* want.

I call it "ugly honesty"—the things that you know deep down but that don't sound or look pretty. Like achieving my mother's ultimate goal for myself, only to realize I really do not enjoy being a stay-at-home mom. I love to work, I love running a business, I care very little for the day-to-day tasks of full-time parenting. Yes, that work is hard and amazing and can be fulfilling, but it is just not the task for me. I don't feel like my best self when that's my only role. I had to admit to myself that when I achieved the thing my mother had wanted her whole life, I found out that it wasn't *my* dream; it was one I adopted from her.

Choosing to lead a life that looks very different from the

one that my parents chose has created friction in our relationship. People are scared of what they don't know, so there was strife when Brady and I decided we wanted to move forty-five minutes away from them into the country. They thought it was an awful idea and that we'd be miserable. They disagreed with the medical choices we made for our kids, with our food and lifestyle choices. Because I was the first of their children to have children and because I chose such a radically different way to raise them, they used our relationship to learn and test the boundaries of being grandparents and being parents to adults. As the oldest, I have always been the one to pave the way for my siblings. I have thick skin—things don't affect me the way they do my brothers and sisters, so if someone has to take the brunt of the strife and disapproval, I am happy to be the one to do it.

It's an understatement to say we've had disagreements; there have been harsh words uttered and arguments had, but we always find a way to get through our differences, agree to disagree, and move forward in the end. Over time, more grandchildren have been added, and my parents have relinquished a lot of their desire for control. They have also mellowed; they're no longer so quick to anger, and they are doting, devoted grandparents who love to spoil their grandkids. Ultimately, I am grateful for our differences and our desire to continue to love and forge a relationship with each other in spite of them.

Nearly from the conception of Instant Loss, I was making as much or more money than Brady every month. Early on in the growth stage of Instant Loss, we began to discuss the possibility that he might come home so we could reverse roles. The way we'd structured our family didn't work with two full-time working parents. Something had to give—it was his job, my job, or the work we were doing homeschooling our kids.

Yes, homeschooling. I have a love-hate relationship with homeschooling. Because of my experience—being pulled out of traditional school, which I loved, when I was in seventh grade, then not receiving further education until college—I swore I'd never homeschool my own children. (Remember what I said about telling God what you won't do?) The power of holding your children's education in your hands always intimidated me. I didn't want to mess it up. I wanted them to have the most opportunities and the best foundation possible. Our kids were young, so we had time to figure out what we were going to do. We ultimately decided we'd cross that bridge when we came to it.

When Avey turned four, it was time to cross the bridge. At that point, I couldn't even imagine parting with one of my babies. They were so young and impressionable. My view on homeschooling began to change and I decided that I would take it a year at a time. So I taught preschool, then kindergarten at home.

Part of parenthood is looking back at the pitfalls and triumphs of your own childhood and deciding which experiences to incorporate into your children's lives and which to leave behind. I never thought I'd end up homeschooling, but it's been an incredibly positive experience for our family. With a mixture of government-approved curriculum, practical skill building, and even a little unschooling, we've discovered the best approach to educating our family.

During Avey's first-grade year, things began to get more chaotic with our schedules. Because of the chaos, we decided that if I could make more income than Brady for six months in a row, he would step down from his position at work. His thought process was that he had a degree so he could always go back to engineering, but I had been presented with a once-in-a-lifetime opportunity. He wanted me to explore it and all the places it could take me.

We also began to consider selling our San Diego home and buying something farther out that was less expensive. Since we would no longer be tied to an office anymore, this was possible. I was also hoping to reduce our monthly expenses as much as we could, since my income wasn't as reliable as Brady's. So we sold our house and relocated to the outskirts of the Southern California desert where we found a magical fifteen-acre plot on the cheap.

When we left Texas, I told Brady we could live anywhere in California but I wouldn't go to the desert. Yet in January 2018, we moved to the desert—another never. Isn't God funny like that?

I'll never be a working mom.

I'll never homeschool.

I'll never move back to California.

I'll never buy a house in the desert.

And here I was, living a life completely composed of nevers. Slowly, it seemed, God was showing me how to love and be open to the wild possibilities that existed beyond my comfort zone. He showed me how to love things I held grave prejudices against and healed the hurt that had led me to hold each prejudice in the first place.

I've learned never to tell God never, to enter into difficult seasons with an open mind and heart that is soft and readied with fertile soil. That way, I can choose to bloom where I'm planted, even if that place looks different from what I had planned for or dreamed of. I've learned that in those places, we often realize that what we picked for ourselves holds merely a fraction of the joy and happiness that these mystical and scary pathways can lead us to.

30

Room at the Table

Dear Body,
   Sometimes life naturally directs us down paths
that we were meant for but never expected to take,
so we go along for the ride, not knowing where we'll
end up but trusting that it'll be somewhere good.
We were handed a tremendous gift, one that has
redirected the course of our life. I've chosen not to
question or overanalyze it but to simply accept it
with gratitude.

I was in full-on go mode. I was asked to be so many things
for so many people. I was running on pure adrenaline, fueled
by whole foods, convinced that if I could just keep my head
down and push, this opportunity I had seized might end up
being our ticket out of the rat race and into a life in which
we weren't working to live but truly living and choosing to
work. Crazy, right? I wanted to start my business properly,
lay the foundation for something that would stand the test of

time. The last thing I wanted was to put time and effort into something that was going to splinter and break apart within the first few years.

After my appearance on *GMA*, I began to field messages from literary agents. They're like real estate agents but they facilitate book deals instead of home sales. I received message after message from book agent after book agent and I let my gut lead me to Andy. I knew she was the one straightaway. We just clicked. Andy was confident that, after *GMA* and the publicity my site had been receiving, we could get a cookbook deal, maybe even with one of the Big Five publishers.

I was a newcomer to the publishing world, but being the bookworm I was, with the time I'd spent working at Barnes & Noble, I knew who the big fish in the ocean of publishing were and I set my sights on Random House. When I told Andy, she chuckled and said we'd take it one offer at a time. I'd been receiving offers for several weeks from a wide range of publishers, but the day after I told Andy that I was fishing for Random House, I received an e-mail from, you guessed it, Random House. We signed in November 2017 and my manuscript was due in January 2018. Yes, friends, you read that correctly. That was just two months. Brady was away on a business trip and wasn't due to come home until January 15, which meant that I would be writing a book while juggling all of my other Instant Loss duties, homeschooling, and keeping house. No pressure.

The amount of work I had to get done between that point and the due date of my manuscript seemed insurmountable. I had to deliver 125 recipes and a ten-thousand-word introduction. I'd never written anything in my life that wasn't a song, an Instagram caption, or a blog post. I hadn't advanced beyond seventh-grade English and had taken just a couple of college courses in the subject. But there I was, responsible for writing an entire book on top of managing Instant Loss online solo. After running at a breakneck pace for eight months, I started to crack.

I was allowed to pull thirty recipes off the website, so I had a head start, but I still had ninety-five to develop from scratch in two months. Not only did the recipes need to be vetted by a professional chef/recipe tester, they needed to be preliminarily tested. As a result, I was in the kitchen constantly, feverishly scribbling on notepads as my army of Instant Pots worked overtime. I constantly reassured myself, "This is only for a season; you can do anything for a season." I wasn't allowed to tell anyone about the book deal, so I had to pretend like things were "normal" online, even though I was in a complete frenzy.

Building a business in the public eye is stressful. You want to put your best foot forward, but I was having trouble making that happen. I'd started building Instant Loss with a plate that was already full. As I continued to grow on Instagram, the eyes of the world were watching not just what I ate but how I mothered and what kind of homemaker I was. They were interested in my relationship with Brady, the clothes that I wore, and the products that I bought. If I put on makeup, I was trying too hard; no makeup, and I looked tired and wasn't trying hard enough. As an extrovert and chronic oversharer, I did not see this as a trespass but as a natural progression. Yet I was overwhelmed. I wasn't sleeping. I was wearing too many hats. My people-pleasing tendencies were in constant overdrive.

Aunt Kim always says, "Not everyone deserves the privilege of knowing your story."

Vulnerability gives others new heights from which to hurt you. I've experienced this in a few personal relationships. Yet as I've gotten older, I'm more careful with my friendships, more protective of my story, but that is difficult when your friends' list on Instagram expands from 400 to 170,000.

The internet can be an amazing tool, but it can also be a vicious instrument. By a wide margin, I receive more positive than negative feedback, but after hearing so many positive things, you can become a bit numb to it. This makes the negative feedback stark in contrast, causing it to feel so much more hurtful.

I've had to develop a thick outer shell. I've had to learn how to navigate the waters of political correctness. Suddenly, people were interested in more than recipes, product suggestions, or motivational stories—they wanted to know who I was voting for, what my religious beliefs were, and how they translated into my political agenda. There's this pervasive thought that has poisoned our society: If someone doesn't believe and act in exactly the way you think they should or if they don't hold your same beliefs, they should be canceled, exiled, cast out.

I was raised with the belief that we make room at the table for everyone. I don't care who you voted for, what your religion is, what country you came from, or if you're my complete opposite. I care about your heart—is it good? Are you loving? Are you kind? Are you living to improve and become the best you can be?

We lose a lot of reality in perception. I've learned there are many people out there who think that if you aren't shouting your views from the rooftops, then you don't care. Often, when we begin to use our influence for things that we weren't called to speak about, we dilute our core message. I was not called to be in politics (thank you, Lord); I was called to use my platform to deliver a message of hope and healing that reveals all we stand to gain when we have faith in ourselves and see the beauty and potential in our own imperfect lives.

I've been told that, as an influencer, I have an obligation to share on every issue that enters our cultural conversation or dominates the news cycle. But that's not the truth. My only obligation is to the Lord and operating within the perimeters He's set. That doesn't mean that I don't care; it doesn't mean that I don't think or pray or cry or scream and rail about it. It doesn't mean that I don't donate or rally my friends. Scripture encourages us not to boast about the good we do in public, to keep it private, because we are storing up our treasures in heaven. I truly believe that prayer and action are much more powerful when we're doing it not to signal virtue to others but because it's what's right.

But there is one topic that I usually receive more hate about than any other: my decision to have skin-removal surgery after my weight loss.

Skin-removal surgery had never been a part of my overall weight-loss plan. To be honest, I never thought about it, and once I lost the weight, the extra skin didn't bother me all that much. It was a by-product of the best thing I'd ever done for myself. I never saw it as a burden or an ugly reminder of the person I once was. I saw it as a badge of honor—my daily prompt to appreciate that I'd done something great.

However, as time went on, I couldn't deny that the excess skin was causing physical problems. I constantly battled rashes, blisters, and sores where the skin folded. I was unable to run or do any kind of rigorous exercise unless the skin was firmly held in place by compression garments. I was also still dealing with issues from my rapid succession of pregnancies that kept me in pain nearly constantly. I had severe abdominal separation and a bladder prolapse that I had been seeing a physical therapist for a couple years to correct. I'd had terrible back pain even before I had Avey. All the doctors I spoke to told me it was because I was overweight, but once I lost the weight, the pain remained. Eventually, my physical therapist told me that repairing the damage that had been done to my muscles was going to require surgery. He suggested an abdominoplasty with muscle repair. While it's commonly referred to as a tummy tuck, it's really a surgical repair for diastasis recti. He even remarked, "This surgery makes extra sense for you because you have all this extra skin."

I went back and forth for half a year. As holistic as I am, I had a deep-seated need to try holistic remedies first: food and exercise cures, natural salves, essential oils, herbs, fascia blasters, garments; surgery just seemed so extreme. My PT said, "Those holistic remedies paired with exercises is what we've been doing for the last two years. It's time." But I was nervous about electing to have surgery. I was even more nervous about sharing it with the world. I knew I'd face harsh criticism and forever be at the mercy of people's assumptions.

I'd heard horror stories about the surgery. Botched jobs, pain-filled recoveries, and more. The closer I came to surgery day, the more dread and anxiety I felt. This was fueled largely by a lot of women who messaged me online and said things like "My sister's husband's friend had that surgery and she said it was the most painful thing she ever did! Good luck with that!"

The night before the surgery, I jokingly asked Brady if I could back out. He smiled and said jokingly that we'd already paid, so there was no turning back now.

I said, "I'm scared. What if this makes things worse?"

"What if it makes it all better?" he replied.

The surgery was a breeze, and the recovery was simple. Having had four C-sections, I knew what healing from abdominal surgery felt like, and this pain was far less than that. The day after surgery, my grandma came to visit. When she rang the doorbell, I opened the front door. She almost fell over in shock.

"What are you doing out of bed?" she exclaimed.

"I feel fine!" I said. "Better than I have in years!"

The back pain had vanished. I didn't even need to take any pain meds past day four. I dealt with swelling on and off for about eighteen months, but I was able to start running five or six months post-op. That's when I began to think about the loose skin that I had on my legs and back.

I wanted to let myself heal for two whole years before I made any decisions about additional surgeries. I wanted to make sure I did my research and that I wasn't catching the "plastics bug." The issues with rashes, tugging, and pulling still persisted in those other areas of my body, but it would be years before I made my ultimate decision about how to handle them. What it really came down to was how incredible my first skin removal surgery experience had been. If it hadn't been so easy, I don't know that I would have felt compelled to address the rest of my body.

As the years went on, my need for the validation and approval of others began to fade. In 2020, I proudly announced that I was going to finish my skin-removal surgeries. I no longer felt the need to overexplain or make excuses. I simply said that I was making this choice because it was what I wanted to do, and you know what? Not a single person messaged me negatively. I believe this is because we teach people how to treat us.

There is a belief on social media that just because you put your life out there and exist, people have the right to tear you down, but I don't condone or accept that. Having access to me is a privilege and if you don't respect that, then you don't deserve that privilege. And it's not just me; this goes for all the people out there who are putting themselves on the line in order to help, inspire, motivate, champion, love, instruct, and share with a passion and vulnerability that are all too rare these days. We should be encouraging these individuals, not trying to diminish them.

People online have watched me grow and develop over the years—in my twenties I tried so hard to be lovable and likable, and as I learned to find my voice blogging, I modeled myself on other influencers; my goal was to be liked, but I wasn't necessarily being authentic. In my thirties, when the fun, mad, crazy, colorful, mystic wanderer in me spilled out, people wondered why I had changed. But I hadn't changed at all; I was just finally letting them in.

31

Community

Dear Body,

Over the past thirty-three years, we have navigated
the beauty and the tragedy of life, breaking wide
open into the woman that we were meant to become.
Together we will continue to mature and develop as
we face what lies ahead. There will be sorrow and grief,
triumph and bliss, and mundane moments that add
balance to it all. I feel truly honored and grateful to still
be here, privileged that I get to continue to experience
all of the intricacies of life. I'm excited for the future
and I can't wait to see what happens next.

I come to consciousness slowly, first becoming aware of the
feel of Brady's stockinged feet resting against mine. It is still
dark outside, maybe four thirty A.M., and the house is calm
and quiet. I'm tempted to stay beneath the covers, feeling the
chill beyond them this winter morning, but my mind is ready
to start the day.

Many things have changed since I made that crazy, wonderful New Year's resolution six years ago to cook every dinner at home. One of the things that surprised me most was that I became a morning person. An insomniac since I was a child, I just thought it was my personality to be a night owl, but it ended up being yet another indicator that I was deeply out of sync with my body. Beginning to respect what my body needed when it came to food led to a cascade of physical healing. My innate internal process that helps guide my body's daily sleep and wake patterns, known as the circadian rhythm, aligned with the sun's waking and setting. Now my internal clock naturally wakes me just before sunrise, and I start to feel tired and ready for bed shortly after it sets.

I sit up on the side of the bed and stretch for a few minutes before making my way to the bathroom. When I come back out, I see the color orange starting to form in a small band just beyond the mountain. It catches my eye through the window, and I toss on my bathrobe, gather my phone, schedule book, pen, and stainless-steel water bottle, and tiptoe downstairs. Tikka, our family dog, gets up to follow me and we both head outside to watch the sunrise. Letting my eyes adjust to the first morning light before looking at a screen makes me feel calm. I plant my bare feet in the dirt, a practice called grounding. I breathe deeply, eyes on the horizon, and rejoice in the dawn for a moment before setting up in my usual spot to check my e-mail. I usually begin work early so I can finish around two P.M. I'm not always perfect at keeping boundaries—it's difficult when what you do for a living blurs the lines between work and home life—but I've been getting better at prioritizing time for work and time for family. Now that my kids are hitting their preteen years, they require more of my emotional and mental support throughout the day.

I research an upcoming blog post that I'll be writing soon,

edit the newsletter, and review a photo and caption that I plan to post that day. I spend hours answering questions, connecting with people, offering support and encouraging words when needed, and before I know it, the sun has risen fully. "Good morning, sun, let's make today count," I say and I gather my things and head back inside.

It's now eight A.M. and the house is abuzz with children talking loudly and classical guitar music that Brady is listening to while doing the dishes from the night before. I catch Brady up on what I need to accomplish for the day while helping with smoothies and pancakes for breakfast. In between, I talk to friends on Instagram as I show them what we're making and link recipes, then retreat upstairs to get in a morning run on the treadmill. It's not lost on me how blessed we are to be living what we love. Things with Instant Loss are as busy as ever, but it's built now, and, to some extent, I have the ability to decide when I work and when I don't. Don't get me wrong—writing four books in five years and continuing to offer free online support and recipes keeps me working a steady five A.M. to two P.M., but I love what I do. It gives me a sense of purpose and drives me to continue to create and to stay open, vulnerable, and honest. And it keeps me connected to you!

One of the pillars of health is community. Our social environments can affect us just as much if not more than our physical environments. When you surround yourself with people who are working toward a similar goal as you—in this case, healthy living—it tends to have a motivating effect. If you watch someone you are in community with have success, it's easier to believe that you can do it too. Obstacles that used to stand in your way become little hurdles to overcome, but you now have a sounding board, a group where you can ask questions and receive advice. Lack of support in relationships is linked to chronic loneliness, which can produce long-term damage to mental health through increased stress hormones and weaker immunity; it can even affect your cardiovascular health.

After my run, I refuel and rehydrate. My family's diet has changed little over the years, though we've slowly cut down on the amount of animal foods and dairy that we eat. Over the past six years, my family went from having a diet that was about 70 percent plant-based to one that is about 90 percent plant-based. We have seen our health improve even further. My cholesterol has decreased, my brain fog has cleared, I no longer feel tired after meals, my energy has doubled, and my blood pressure is the best it's ever been! A plant-based diet minimizes intake of processed foods, meat, eggs, and dairy and maximizes the consumption of plant foods, like fruits, vegetables, legumes, nuts and seeds, whole grains, mushrooms, herbs, and spices. This is the only diet on record proven to reverse heart disease in the majority of patients, repairing and opening arteries without surgery or drugs. It's no coincidence that, according to a study published in March 2017 in *Nutrition and Diabetes,* people who followed this diet lost more weight at six and twelve months than people who followed any other diet that did not limit calories or require regular exercise. (I'm such an advocate for this way of eating that in 2019 I won the American Heart Association's Lifestyle Change Award and spoke at their annual conference—it was one of the greatest honors of my life.)

I used to view eating well as simply a tool for weight loss, but now I utilize it as a tool to keep me healthy. I *feel* so much healthier that it encourages me to continue on this path; it doesn't hurt that the food is outstanding. My thyroid disease is in remission, and I've been off medication for six years. My keratosis pilaris has cleared up, my restless legs syndrome and insomnia are both gone, and I've seen a vast improvement in my mental health, hormonal cycles, energy levels, and immune function. Our bodies send us all kinds of signals when something isn't working for us; we just need to listen.

I no longer feel like I have no control over my body; my body and I work in tandem to create our highest quality of life. Permanent weight loss requires permanent dietary changes. (Not to imply that I am absolutely adherent to them all the time . . . which I'll talk about more in a bit.) My healthier habits have become a way of life. But in order to make them last, I had to create something that was sustainable not only for me, but for my family.

Just because a diet is effective does not mean that it's sustainable. Diets only work if people stick with them. Any diet that reduces caloric intake can result in weight loss. But taking the pounds off doesn't seem to be the biggest issue for anyone, myself included. The hardest part is keeping them off. Part of my success maintaining comes from a mindset of abundance, not of restriction; instead of looking at all the things I shouldn't eat, I focus on what I should and on all the miraculous benefits of those foods that reach far beyond weight loss. I consume as many fibrous vegetables and fruits as I want.

In the beginning, I leaned on the Arizona State University School for Health and Nutrition for their portion guidelines. I kept animal-protein sources to about the size of my palm, fats to the size of my thumb (except for peanut butter—that deserves to be doubled), and starchy carbohydrates to the size of a clenched fist. I didn't count points or macros; I simply trusted my body to self-regulate, much like a child's body does before hyperpalatable foods and negative adult input, like forcing foods at mealtime "or else," interfere with that natural regulation. I focus on the quality of our food and all of those incredible micronutrients, not their calorie count (which often isn't accurate anyway). It's not about what you eat but what you absorb. Vegetarians who consume the same amount of calories or as much as four hundred more than nonvegetarians lose more weight and maintain their weight because of their higher resting metabolic rate. It's been widely known for more than thirty years that those who eat primarily plant-based foods weigh about twenty to thirty pounds less than the general population. The more plant-based foods people eat, the lower their weight seems to be.

When I embarked on this journey, I learned as I went. I didn't have all of the answers—I don't even have them all now—but I started where I was. I began to change the environment of my home to facilitate the changes I wanted to see. I continue to learn as I go; I read books and studies, watch documentaries, and listen to podcasts. I know that to build on this, I need to nurture that growth mindset. I also feel the weight of responsibility for a community that trusts me to continue to be encouraging and provide new information to support the things that I'm doing for my family.

It is not something that I take lightly.

We are all biologically individual, which explains why some of us feel better consuming plant-based diets and others feel their best with animal-based diets. This is something that you are going to have to discover for yourself. There is one thing that everyone agrees on, though: Plant foods are essential, and they should make up the bulk of your nutrition. Regardless of how you choose to eat, I support you and commend you for putting thought and effort into prioritizing your health and the health of your family. It certainly isn't easy in this toxic food environment that we live in, but the more we change, the more we'll see change in that regard.

Solidly in maintenance and past the five-year weight-loss

mark, I feel like I've found the key not just to weight loss but to happiness in general. There is a meme that I love, a little drawing of a critter holding a jar that says HAPPINESS on it. Someone off the page asks, "Where did you get that?" And the critter replies, "I made it myself."

The Bible says that joy comes from the Lord, but I believe that happiness is something you cultivate yourself. I felt stuck in my life for a long time; it was only when I stepped out in courage and decided to change it that something really meaningful happened. I think there is a lot to be said for ownership. The bad news is that you've got to change, but the good news is that you have the power to change, and when you realize you have the power to achieve your goals, the whole world opens up for you. I began to work toward the life that I wanted, and slowly it became the life that I always dreamed about. It still doesn't look like everything that I envisioned—I don't know that it will this side of heaven—but I truly feel that I could not ask for more.

For lunch, I make a sprouted three-bean chili and corn bread, and we all sit together at our dining-room table and talk about the day so far and the hiking trip we've planned for the upcoming weekend. We've become quite the active bunch, national park–hopping, exploring rural places in our van, and logging thousands of miles on the road. I discovered my love for hiking after we moved out to the desert. Dozens of trails surround our house and I have miles and miles of naked desert to explore every day, something I take full advantage of. Most days it's my reward for working in front of a screen for hours on end. The benefits of walking and hiking are immense. My physician told me years ago that she could prescribe me either an antidepressant or thirty minutes of activity a day; she told me that they both have the same effect on the brain. I opted for the activity and miraculously haven't struggled with depression since 2016. I am not saying that this will be the case for everyone, but it certainly helped me. When I'm active, I experience fewer bouts of anxiety. I get that runners' high that everyone talks about. It really is nature's antidepressant.

The more in tune I've become with my body, the more fine-tuned my diet has become. Getting rid of the chronic inflammation made it possible for me to tap into exactly how my body feels after each meal, each run, each hike, and keeps me pressing to optimize what makes her feel best. Please don't get me wrong—I still battle demons. I have had regains of about thirty pounds a couple different times and frequent fluctuations of about ten to fifteen pounds. I love the lifestyle that I've created, and there is nothing on earth that makes me feel quite as amazing, but that's not to say that I don't still struggle with self-sabotaging behaviors or try to run and hide from emotions that feel too big and scary. It's easy for me to go back to trying to cover them up with food. But doing so never takes me to a good place; self-medicating always reminds me why I don't self-medicate anymore: It never solves anything, but it does make a lot of things worse.

I try to respect myself and my body. I don't like it when she feels sick, and I hate that I'm the one who causes it. Every year, it gets a little easier. I learn a little bit more. The foods of my past hold a little less appeal. One day, I'm hopeful that I will have completely overcome these behaviors that used to be constant and have now become rare. But if I never do, I am grateful for that as well, because every time I fall, I am reminded why it's important to keep going, what I stand to lose because of all that I've gained. This propels me forward. Not always immediately—I've been known to sit and wallow;

I give space for that too—but eventually I get up, own it, and move forward.

After lunch, I march back upstairs to edit video content and answer more messages. The stream of comments is constant now, never ending. I couldn't get to the bottom of them even if I hired full-time help, and that's okay. I've made peace with the fact that I won't be able to respond to everyone, but I feel it's important that I'm the one who continues to answer, not a team of outside people. I trust that the messages I'm supposed to answer will be ones that find me throughout the day, and with the rest, I ask for grace. And I'm not saying this to discourage anyone from dropping me a line—truly, conversing with you is the best part of what I do.

Around two thirty P.M., I officially tap out. I will still continue to answer messages and post stories until I head to bed, but my official workday has ended and I poke my head into Brady's shop to find him working on a table he's building. "Want to walk?" I ask, moving my eyebrows up and down.

He smiles. "Sure thing. Let me finish up here and change my shoes."

I head back into the house and get caught up in a conversation with Avey, our resident chatterbox. Built like her mama, she goes on and on about a dream she had, then a friend she's been hanging out with lately, and then she jumps to asking me about the first boy I liked and my first kiss. We have certainly moved into a different season of life, and I can't believe that she's almost a teenager. Arthritis flare-ups haven't plagued her in years and for the most part we've been able to keep her disease under control with diet and environment. There have been times when we've had to go back on medicine and I'm thankful that we have the ability to use all of these things to facilitate her best quality of life.

I ask the boys if they want to hike with us, but they're

caught up in a board game and opt to stay behind. "Looks like it's just you and me," I say to Brady as I grab my jacket and his hand on the way out the door.

"Eh, I like it that way anyway," he replies and gives my hand a squeeze.

The years have been kind to us; we have twelve years of marriage under our belts and a lifetime's worth of life experience. We feel older than we are; in a way, we always have. I can honestly say he is still my very best friend. It hasn't been a storybook romance, but it's been real and ours, and I would never trade it.

There are times when we get on each other's nerves, of course, times when we don't agree or see eye to eye, but something we are very diligent about is prioritizing our relationship over just about everything else. I've become less codependent and more interdependent, which has relieved the burden on us both, and Brady is becoming a better communicator every day. What we learned in premarital counseling all those years ago is something we still carry with us—that the number-one reason why marriages end in divorce is unmet expectations. So we talk about expectations a lot and how we can better meet them or adjust them in order to alleviate tension or communicate care and love in better ways. I feel like this has truly been a foundational thing for us and one reason why we were able to pull through difficult times and move forward.

After we get back home, we dive into making dinner. Tostadas are a household favorite and easy enough to throw together. Brady makes the tortillas from scratch as I work on the beans and vegetables to go on top. We field questions from the kids as we work in tandem, and the house feels warm with love and light.

This is not an ending but rather the bookmark of a new

beginning. In life, we start over a thousand times. Every mis-step, failure, or roadblock is not a stopping point; it's a chance to learn, grow, and begin again. We will always have new lessons to learn, stories to tell, and roads to walk, some bumpier than others. But I have found that they will always lead us somewhere good, if we let them.

I was just a girl who lost a hundred and twenty-five pounds, but the focus shouldn't be on what I lost, but who I became.

Dear Friend

Instant Loss was a passion project. There was no guarantee it would work out, but I poured every ounce of myself into it. I was willing to work hard, harder than I'd ever worked in my life. I was willing to lose sleep; I was willing to work for free until I had a product people were willing to buy. I put in hundreds of unpaid hours, maybe thousands—and I still do. Because it's not about the money; it's about the people. I was willing to be wrong. I was willing to be corrected. I was willing to learn as I went, willing to fake it till I made it while also being vulnerable enough to share with the world that I was really just learning as I went along (isn't everyone?).

Now the number-one question I receive is "But how?"

"How do I start?"

"How do I nurture my body and lose the weight?"

"I've tried and tried and tried—why don't I succeed?"

The truth is, many of us have been dieting for long enough that we have basic food knowledge. We know to eat vegetables and that the healthiest people in the world have a more plant-based diet. We know about macronutrients, that we need to balance carbohydrate intake with fat intake, and that we should consume adequate amounts of protein. What many people don't know, however, is how to practice the consistency, patience, and perseverance required to go the distance and obtain the ultimate wellness we're striving for. Remember, it's not about achieving perfection; it's about reaching a point where your body is operating at peak wellness, and this occurs only after you can be consistent for days, then weeks, then months, then years.

As you work toward your goals, you'll discover that this is an exercise more for your psyche than anything else. Maya Angelou said, "Forgive yourself for not knowing what you didn't know before you learned it." It's all about learning to honor your body and prioritizing its needs over your fleeting desires. Many of us have never practiced this before. It's like an atrophied muscle you have to strengthen. I've said it a million times, but it really started to click for me when I began to treat my body like she's a toddler.

I'm a mama, I know how to care for one of those.

I make sure she drinks enough water; I put her to bed at bedtime; I tell her she can't have twelve cookies; I make sure she finishes her vegetables; I remind her how smart she is; I tell her how kind she is; I make sure she knows how important she is.

At first, it might feel all-consuming. It's going to take up a lot of brain space as you adjust to a new plan and try to navigate withdrawal from processed foods. That part lasts about three weeks if you're starting for the first time, and that is where perseverance is essential. If you're a chronic overeater, that's also the period in which your stomach will begin to adjust and feel satisfied with healthier portion sizes.

You might experience resistance from loved ones at first— food pushers at holidays who insist you eat things you've politely declined, spouses who aren't fully on board, friends who tell you that it's not possible. Gather close to you the people who believe in and support your vision, and push those who don't to the periphery. Our environment really does dictate our success; this is why it's crucial to alter not only your diet but your environment. Find a group of people who are on the same path as you, lean on them, learn from them, and create new patterns and behaviors together. Lean into your faith, whatever that means to you—faith in yourself, faith in a higher power. For me, being able to trust that God was directing my steps in the midst of uncertainty helped keep me on track.

I know it's a lot to tackle, and I'm not going to pull any punches: *It's hard.*

And in a world where people value comfort and "feel good" more than they value health, it's natural to resist the discomfort. But like they say, life begins at the end of your comfort zone. Where there is no struggle, there is no strength. It's hard to leave comfort behind, but you have to let go of the life you're familiar with to live the life you've always dreamed about.

You can. You will.

And this is your jumping-off point.

ACKNOWLEDGMENTS

I've started writing this page dozens of times. I want to get it right because to me it's the most important page in this book. Enduring what I've endured and accomplishing what I've accomplished have amplified my appreciation for life.

Gratitude is as essential to me as breathing. I have been filled with understanding that I pray deepens, compassion that I pray expands, and a thankfulness so immense I pray it never leaves or lessens.

Will Arnett says, "I am happy because I am grateful. I choose to be grateful. That gratitude allows me to be happy."

Who am I to write a book? Have these opportunities? Meet the people that I have? Live this life full of abundance that I've been given? There are so many who are more deserving. My suffering pales in comparison to the suffering of others. My triumphs are only triumphant because of better people than I, and God of course, always God. I do not hold the answers to these questions, but I do hold a tremendous amount of gratitude to those who have helped to teach me, shape me, and provide me with opportunities I never dreamed I'd have.

To Brady, how to begin to say thank you? When I started praying for you all those years ago, I asked for a best friend, but I didn't fully understand what I was requesting. Someone who carries you to bed when you can't move from surgery or from grief. Someone who knows the best and the worst of you and loves the dark just as much as the light. The keeper of my confidence, the father of my babies, the one who keeps the house warm because I won't touch the thermostat, and gets food in my belly when I'm too busy working to pause to eat.

You carry us all. In good times and in bad and you never complain. You're the hardest worker I've ever met and there isn't a thing you can't fix: air fryers, toilets, cars, even me. You've helped heal me in a hundred different ways since we met; you've broken me wide open too, but I think that was important as well.

I'm grateful that the worst things that have ever happened to us have become part of a greater story and that in the face of some of life's biggest trials we chose each other, our family, and to fix it instead of throw it away.

You're good at fixing things and I like to think I've picked up a little of that through watching you. Thank you for rubbing my bottom at night, telling me all the reasons why you love me and inventing new ones anytime I ask, for making me laugh harder than anyone ever has, and for letting me share some of our secrets.

There's no one else like you; you're one of the good ones.

My kids, full of wonder and adventure, you take me back to places I haven't known since I was a child. I am so lucky to have you, and I'm so proud of the people you are becoming. Your fearless nature, your honest hearts, and your kindness will take you far. Thank you for sharing me with the world; I'm so grateful to be able to do both.

My parents, you were and are wonderful parents. I'm glad that in spite of our differences we continue to love one another and prioritize our relationship. I believe that it is due in part to your unwavering belief in me that I was able to accomplish all that I have. I love you.

Acknowledgments

My siblings, thank you for being my peers and teachers. For the after-work phone calls, the countless memes and song threads, and for not just being the family I was given but the one I choose. Love you guys.

My grandparents, ever faithful angels on my shoulders guiding me gently, imparting wisdom and love—I am so lucky to have you.

Aunt Kim, older sister, mentor, friend—you are many things to me, and I think that is exactly what aunts were meant to be: unassuming heroes that fit into whatever role you need them to play, waiting in the wings to provide you with advice born from life experience and lessons earned. You planted the seeds and I have enjoyed the harvest. I am immeasurably grateful for you.

My friends, too many to name so I won't list you all, but you know who you are . . . my comic relief, amateur detectives-in-arms, sisters who know me better than I know myself. This book would not have been possible without your support. I forever love you.

My agent, Andy, the day you slid into my DMs was truly heaven sent. I can't believe we conquered another one. There were times I never thought we'd make it through this guy, he was a beast to write, but I'm glad we stuck it out through thick and thin. Don't know how I'd manage without you, or I do, it just wouldn't be very pretty.

My editors, Sarah and Amanda, Lord knows this book would not have been possible without you. Thank you for being my teachers, giving assignments to this novice writer who really had no business writing anything at all. Thank you for taking me under your wing, teasing out all the good bits, and policing my runaway thought patterns. If this book is any good at all it's only because of the two of you. I appreciate you, I love you, thank you.

Acknowledgments

Photography team, Vanessa, Chris, and Luca, and the art team at HarperCollins, thank you for helping us create such a spectacular cover. It was everything I envisioned and more!

HarperCollins team, thank you for giving me the opportunity to write this story. Thank you for believing in it and helping me share it.

God, thank you for letting me dream wild, crazy, tremendous dreams and directing my steps as I venture into the unknown time and time again. Nothing is unknown to You.